The Science of Eating Raw

How to Lose Weight, Increase Your Energy, Prevent Disease, & Meet All of Your Nutritional Needs on a Raw Food Diet

By Swayze Foster

Disclaimer

The information provided in this book is intended to provide helpful information on eating a healthy raw food diet. This book is not meant to be used, nor should it be used, to diagnose or treat any medical condition. For diagnosis or treatment of any medical problem, consult your own physician.

The author is not responsible for any specific health or allergy needs that may require medical supervision and is not liable for any damages or negative consequences from any treatment, action, application or preparation, to any person reading or following the information in this book. References are provided for informational purposes only and do not constitute endorsement of any websites or other sources. Readers should be aware that the websites listed in this book may change.

To Mom, Dad, and Daximus

CONTENTS

Introduction

How would you like to avoid—and in many cases even reverse— the now common diseases that are killing millions of people each year like heart disease, stroke, cancer, and type II diabetes?

You can with a healthy and sustainable raw food diet.

How would you also like to avoid all of the common non-life-threatening diseases such as colds, flus, allergies, headaches, migraines, and joint pains?

Yep, a raw food lifestyle can offer that too.

How would you like to experience much more energy and mental clarity without coffee, sodas, energy drinks, or other unhealthy stimulants?

That's right, raw foods again. And I'm not done yet...

How would you like to lose excess fat and reach your ideal weight, not for the next few weeks or months, but for the rest of your life?

You've got it, a raw food diet wins again! And I think it's safe to say that virtually every person on the planet wants these things for themselves.

No one wants to suffer and die from cancer. No one likes getting runny noses or sore throats when the weather changes. No one wants to rely on cup after cup of coffee to keep from falling face-first onto their keyboards.

And of course, no one wants to remain fat and unattractive. We all want sexy slim physiques so we can feel proud of the way we look and garner the attention of other sexy slim guys and gals.

We also want clear skin, great hair, strong nails, healthy teeth, and just an overall sense of wellbeing and happiness.

A raw food diet can provide all of this and more. But not just *any* raw food diet...

The Raw Food Movement Needs a Facelift

For far too long, the message from many raw food leaders has been "Cut out cooked foods, eat raw, and voila!" Sorry dear reader, but it's a bit more complicated than that.

Sure, a lot of people experience tremendous health improvements simply by cutting out cooked foods and gobbling up any raw foods in any amounts they please. But this isn't a good long-term strategy. Eating a 100% raw diet does not guarantee nutritional sufficiency.

Yes, malnutrition is possible on a raw food diet. In fact, it's probable if you follow 99% of raw food plans available today!

My goal in writing this book—besides selling a billion copies and making beaucoup bucks, of course—is to teach you all you need to know about thriving with a raw food lifestyle in today's modern, non-raw world.

It's simpler and easier than you may think.

The Science of Eating Raw

My other goal in writing this book has to do with one small but oh-so important word: science.

You see, most books on the whys of raw food feasting use pseudoscientific gobbledygook to back up their claims. As you'll soon learn, plant enzymes, digestive leukocytosis, and the ever-popular exclamation "All wild animals eat raw so we should too!" are not good reasons to adopt a raw food diet.

In *The Science of Eating Raw*, I've included hundreds of scientific references to back up my claims. You'll learn the real whys of eating a raw vegan diet—the science-based whys—so that you will be in complete control of your health and lifestyle.

No more hemming and hawing or changing the subject when someone asks you "Where do you get your protein?" or "What about B12?" or "Don't you know a raw food diet will leak you weak and toothless?".

No more turning to raw food gurus for "necessary" recipes and menu plans. This book will show you how to create raw recipes and meal plans that are delicious, satisfying, and packed with nutrition.

In a nutshell, *The Science of Eating Raw* will show you what to do and why to do it so you can finally achieve and maintain the awesome health and fitness results you've been searching for.

Sound good? Great, let's do this!

But first, a little bit about me and my raw food journey...

My (Very) Short Story

Since this book is all about helping YOU go raw and get healthy, I won't regale you with a longwinded recount of my personal history with raw foods. Suffice it to say that before adopting a raw food diet, I wasn't healthy nor was I happy.

Anemia kept me drained of energy and made driving to school and work a danger to myself and others.

Restless leg syndrome (RLS) kept me fidgety and uncomfortable while attempting to sit still or fall asleep at night.

Frequent knee pain kept me from doing the activities I loved, like step aerobics (don't laugh).

Seasonal colds kept my nose runny and my throat sore four times a year.

Heavy menstrual cycles kept me bloated and in pain for a full week each month.

Keratosis pilaris (chicken skin) and back acne kept me frustrated and embarrassed about my body.

7

Constant dieting to keep unwanted weight off kept me craving more food. Cravings inevitably led to bingeing and purging, which left me feeling guilty and ashamed.

All of this at just 19 years old AND while eating a supposedly healthy cooked vegan diet!

When I adopted a low fat raw food lifestyle in 2007, everything changed. No more anemia, no more restless leg syndrome, no more seemingly inexplicable joint pain, no more colds, no more unbearable periods and no more red and bumpy skin.

It was incredibly liberating, but that's not to say things were perfect. I made many mistakes—some for many months and some that were quite serious and even life-threatening in the long run—that kept me from having the energy, body, and piece of mind that I desired.

Once I FINALLY figured out that my problems were simply due to eating an insufficient diet, I made a change in the way I was eating raw. Almost immediately, my cravings disappeared, my energy went through the roof, and I achieved my best body WITHOUT calorie restriction.

As I already said, my goal in writing *The Science of Eating Raw* is to teach you how to thrive on a raw food diet. This means avoiding the many mistakes that I made so you can start out on the right foot.

So Are You Ready?

Are you ready to go raw so you can experience the best body, energy, digestion, and overall wellbeing of your life?

Yes? Then turn the page and let's begin!

CHAPTER 1
Why Vegan?

Why vegan? Because it's healthier, plain and simple.

Don't believe me? Let's check out the facts.

The China Study

The China Project (or China Study), conducted in 1983, looked at 6,500 men and women from 65 counties in China. Blood and urine samples from each person were analyzed and questionnaires administered. In addition, the diet of each person and his or her family was monitored for three days and food samples from marketplaces across China were taken for analysis.[1]

The findings?

The researchers found a very strong correlation between meat, dairy, and egg consumption and cancer. It went something like this: the more animal products consumed, the higher the risk for cancer.[1]

And I'm not talking about just one type of cancer. I mean colon cancer, lung cancer, breast cancer, prostate cancer, stomach cancer, liver cancer, and also diabetes and heart disease. All of these diseases have been linked to animal and animal by-products in the diet.[1]

And of course, I can't forget about high cholesterol. As Colin T. Campbell writes in *The China Study: Starling Implication for Diet, Weight Loss, and Long-Term Health*:

> At the outset of the China Study, no one could or would have predicted that there would be a relationship between cholesterol and any of the disease rates. What a surprise we got! As blood

9

cholesterol levels decreased from 170 mg/dL to 90 mg/dL, cancers of the liver, rectum, colon, male lung, female lung, breast, childhood leukemia, adult leukemia, childhood brain, adult brain, stomach, and esophagus (throat) decreased.[1]

This means if you want to dramatically cut down on your risk for various types of cancer, you have to severely limit (no more than 10 ounces per week) all meat, milk, eggs, butter, and, yes, even cheese, from your diet.

Still not convinced that animal products are unhealthy? Then let's dig a little deeper...

Meat

Meat—whether it's fatty red meat, "lean" poultry, or grass-fed organic pork—is an unhealthy food for humans.

Fat and Cholesterol

A major downfall of meat is that it's high in fat—saturated fat, the worst kind—and cholesterol, both of which raise cholesterol levels in the body. High cholesterol (hypercholesterolemia) means an increased risk for the number one killer in America: heart disease.[*1-6, 7]

High amounts of saturated fat and cholesterol have also been linked to stroke, type II diabetes, breast cancer, obesity, ovarian cancer, prostate cancer, colorectal cancer, poor cognitive function and memory, and death.[10, 11-12, 13-15, 17-18, 19-21, 22-25, 26-27, 28, 29]

Calories

Because meat is so high in fat, it's also very high in calories. Just 3 ounces of pork shoulder is 69% fat and 200 calories! This means that it is very easy to overeat and gain unwanted weight.

---

[*] Although the American Heart Association advocates a total blood cholesterol level of less than 200 mg/dL, the physicians whose programs consistently get results—like Dr. Caldwell Esselstyn's, Dr. Joel Fuhrman's, and Dr. John McDougall's programs—advocate a total cholesterol below 150 mg/dL and/or an LDL cholesterol below 100 mg/dL.[2, 8, 9]

Even if you don't overeat, you may still find it difficult to maintain a healthy weight while eating meat. One study that assessed 103,455 men and 270,348 women over a 5-year period found that "meat consumption was positively associated with weight gain in women and men, in normal-weight and overweight subjects, and in smokers and non-smokers," *after controlling for total caloric intake!*[30]

So let's say you have two people eating 2,000 calories every day, but one person eats no meat while the other eats 250 grams (9 ounces) every day. Based on the results of this study, the meat-eater would be expected to gain more than 2 kg (4.4 lbs) after 5 years.[30]

Fiber

Another bad thing about meat is that it contains no fiber. A diet high in fiber is absolutely vital for proper digestion and feelings of fullness after a meal.[31-33]

Fiber is also great for boosting good bacteria in our guts.[34] No probiotics necessary.

Alzheimer's, Lung Cancer, and Gout, Oh My!

And it doesn't stop there. Here are just a few more serious illnesses that have been linked to meat consumption:

- Alzheimer's disease[35-36]
- Chronic obstructive pulmonary disease (COPD)[37-40]
- Dementia[41-42]
- Endotoxemia[43-44]
- Esophageal cancer[45-47]
- Gout[48]
- Kidney stones[49-50]
- Liver cancer[47, 51]
- Bone Mineral Density Loss[52-53]
- Lung cancer[47]
- Lukemia[54-55]
- Pancreatic cancer[56-57]
- Rheumatoid arthritis[58-59]
- Stomach cancer[60-62]
- Type I diabetes[63]

Just by removing meat from your diet, you can significantly reduce your risk of developing most of the big-name Western diseases.

Acidity

Your body is always trying to maintain an alkaline state of approximately 7.4 blood pH. Unlike fruits and vegetables, meat is metabolized to acidic compounds due to the high amounts of acid minerals like phosphorus it contains.

In other words, meat is acid-forming.

Eating a diet that's heavy in meat and other acid-forming foods causes metabolic acidosis. To maintain the slightly alkaline state mentioned above, your body must leach alkaline minerals like calcium from your bones, creating a lower bone mineral density.[64-65] Chronic metabolic acidosis also causes muscle loss and even kidney stones.[65-66]

Bacteria

As we all know, meat is subject to various harmful bacteria including e. coli and salmonella. In fact, all of the bacteria and viruses that are responsible for the most illnesses and deaths from food poisoning in the United States are found on meat and other animal products.[67]

Think your meat is bacteria-free because you buy it neatly wrapped from a prominent chain grocery store? Think again.

In a study published in 2005, researchers tested over 1,000 food samples and found that 69% of pork and beef and 92% of poultry were contaminated with fecal matter containing *E. coli*.[68]

While cooking kills off most of these bacteria, cooking meat at high temperatures also produces mutagenic compounds like Heterocyclic amines (HCAs), polycyclic aromatic hydrocarbons (PAHs), and Advanced Glycemic End Products (AGEs).[69-70, 71-72, 73-74]

Antibiotics

Most meats also contain antibiotics. In 2009, close to 80% of antimicrobial drugs produced in the United States were used by factory farmers.[75] This practice, which is done to make the animals grow faster, has some dire long-term consequences. We are already seeing new microorganisms (aka "superbugs") that are resistant to these drugs.[76-79]

And while antibiotic-free meats are available, these meats are not always free from harmful bacteria. Several recent studies have found Methicillin-resistant *Staphylococcus aureus* and *Escherichia coli*, two antibiotic-resistant forms of *E. coli*, and Enterococcus in antibiotic-free pork, beef, and chicken.[80-81]

Other Contaminants

Contamination doesn't end with bacteria and antibiotics. Factory farmed meat also contains synthetic hormones, which may increase the risk for breast cancer and prostate cancer in humans and dioxins, which have been linked to ovarian cancer and kidney disease in mice.[*82, 83-85]

Dairy

Many people learn about the dangers of meat, cut it out of their diet, but keep consuming dairy products like milk, butter, cheese, and yogurt. This is a big mistake for several reasons.

Fat and Cholesterol

Like meat, dairy products are full of fat. Whole milk is 48% fat, cheddar cheese is 73% fat, and butter is almost 100% fat. All three contain lots of artery-clogging cholesterol as well.

Calories

Also like meat, dairy products are high in calories. One cup of whole cow's milk contains almost 150 calories, one ounce of cheddar cheese

---

* Since more than 90% of exposure to dioxins comes from our diet (mainly from meat, dairy, and fish), it's no surprise that a study analyzing the amount of dioxin in various foodstuffs found a "simulated vegan diet" of fruits, vegetables, legumes, and grains to have the lowest amount.[83-84]

is 114 calories, and there are over 100 calories in just one tablespoon of butter!

Fiber

Again like meat, dairy products are completely fiber-free. Say bye-bye to regular bowel movements!

Breast Cancer, Prostate Cancer, and Acne, Oh My!

Below are just a few of the diseases and disorders that have been linked to dairy consumption:

- Acne[86-88]
- Autism[89-90]
- Breast cancer[91]
- Heart disease[92]
- Migraine headaches[93-94]
- Multiple sclerosis[95-96]
- Ovarian cancer[97-99]
- Parkinson's disease[100-101]
- Prostate cancer[91, 102-103]
- Testicular cancer[104]
- Type I diabetes[63, 105-106]

Acidity

Like meat—do I sound like a broken record yet?—dairy products are acid-forming and can lead to bone and muscle loss.

This likely explains why countries with the highest milk consumption also have the most incidences of hip fractures and osteoporosis.[107-108] (For more information on this "calcium paradox," please see chapter six.)

Opiates

Did you know that both cow's milk and human milk contain small amounts of opiates like morphine? Yes, you read that right: morphine is in your milk, your cheese, your ice cream, and your yogurt.

The primary protein in milk is called casein. When casein is broken down via digestion, opiates called casomorphins are released into your body.

Why are casomorphins in cow's milk? In *Breaking the Food Seduction: The Hidden Reasons Behind Food Cravings—-And 7 Steps to End Them Naturally*, Dr. Neal Barnard writes:

> **It appears that the opiates from mother's milk produce a calming effect on the infant and, in fact, may be responsible for a good measure of the mother-infant bond...Like it or not, mother's milk has a druglike [sic] effect on the baby's brain that ensures that the baby will bond with Mom and continue to nurse and get the nutrients all babies need.[109]**

While great for baby cows, these addictive substances were not intended for adult humans (or adult cows, for that matter). In fact, the presence of morphine, codeine, and other opiates may explain why so many people find it more difficult to give up dairy products like milk, cheese, and ice cream than meats like beef, pork, and fish.

Other Contaminants

Like meat, milk also contains antibiotics, hormones, and dioxins. One example is estrogen, a hormone present in large amounts in factory farmed cows that has been linked to early onset puberty in girls.[110-111]

Eggs

Eggs are high in fat, calories and cholesterol, contain no fiber, and are acid-forming when consumed. Egg consumption has been linked to various diseases including type II diabetes, prostate cancer, colorectal cancer and bladder cancer.[112-113, 114, 115-117, 118]

One study found that just 2-4 eggs per week increased the risk for type II diabetes in women by 19%, and 7 or more eggs per week by 77%.[112] Another one found that just 2.5 or more eggs per week increased the risk for developing prostate cancer by 81%![114]

Like meat and milk, eggs are also subject to various contaminants, including bacteria and antibiotics.

What About Fish?

Fish flesh is meat, plain and simple. It's full of fat and cholesterol. It's fiberless and acid-forming just like beef, pork, lamb, and chicken.

Fish are also full of dangerous chemicals like dioxins, polychlorinated biphenyls (PCBs), and methylmercury (MeHg).[84, 119-120, 121] One study found that freshwater fish had the highest levels of dioxins of all foodstuffs that were analyzed, including beef, chicken, pork, butter, and eggs.* **[84]

What About Lean Meat, Skim Milk, and Low-Fat Yogurt?

Just because a food is low in fat does not mean it is a health food. Many hard candies are low in fat, but we certainly wouldn't consider them healthy. Sugar in a bag is also fat-free, but you don't need me to tell you it's junk food.

In any event, low-fat animal products usually aren't really low in fat.

Low-fat milk is a perfect example. Look up 2% milk in any calorie counting database and you'll see that it's actually 35% fat. That's because the 2% refers to the amount of fat by weight, not by calories.

Chicken is another example of misleading marketing. While labeled 98% fat-free, chicken breast is almost 20% fat. Again, the 98% figure refers to the weight, not the calories.

---

* Saltwater fish had significantly lower levels, but were still over four times higher in dioxins than were plant foods.[84]

** Wondering how you can get enough omega-3 fatty acids without fish? Chia seeds, flax seeds, walnuts, and hemp seeds, are all excellent fish-free sources.

The Truth About Lean Deli Meats

For convenience and often in an effort to eat healthier, many people opt for lean deli meats like sliced chicken, turkey, and ham. Unfortunately, these are not health foods.

Deli meats typically contain lots of salt; lots of preservatives like sodium nitrate, a preservative and known carcinogenic precursor; and lots of monosodium glutamate (MSG), a dangerous neurotoxin.[122-123] They're also more likely to be contaminated with the bacteria *Listeria*, which can come in contact with these meats in between the cooking and packaging processes.[124-125]

Finally, an overwhelming number of studies have linked deli meats and other processed meat products to various cancers, including colorectal and prostate cancer.[126-128]

"Low-Fat" Dairy Products

At 35% of calories coming from fat, 2% milk is not really low-fat. Neither is 1% milk, which contains 21% fat. Even the nonfat label is misleading, with "non-fat" milk containing about 2% fat.

Regardless of fat intake, there are plenty of reasons to forgo low-fat dairy products. Just like their whole fat counterpart, these foods are fiberless, acid-forming, and contain unwanted substances like casein, opioids, harmful bacteria, and antibiotics.

But Yogurt is So Good for You!

No, it isn't. Plain, whole milk yogurt is high in calories (138 calories per 8 ounce container), full of fat (47%), contains no fiber, and has been linked to ovarian cancer.[129-132]

Low-fat yogurt isn't much better. In addition to being loaded with sugar and artificial sweeteners, researchers found that women who ate low-fat yogurt once a day were 1.6 times more likely to have children who developed asthma.[133]

What a random piece of info

17

Low-Fat Meat is Still Meat, Low-Fat Milk is Still Milk

"Low-fat" or not, these foods are still animal products. Lean deli meats contain no fiber, are acidic, and often contain unwanted hormones, antibiotics, and bacteria. And "low-fat" milks, cheeses, and yogurts are not free from cholesterol, casein, or opiates like morphine.

But What About Protein?

Contrary to popular opinion, human protein needs are quite small. In actuality, one of the most common dietary mistakes made today is eating too much protein! The human body cannot store extra protein so any excess in your diet must be excreted, which means more work for you kidneys and liver.

Excess animal protein has been linked to all sorts of health problems, including dehydration, cardiovascular disease, osteoporosis, and cancer.[1, 134, 135-136, 137, 138]

What about weight loss? Aren't meat-heavy, high-protein diets like Atkins, Zone, and paleo great for helping you lose weight and get in shape?

Yes, you will likely lose weight quickly on such diets, but at what cost? According to Dr. Joel Fuhrman, author of the popular plant-based diet book *Eat To Live: The Revolutionary Formula for Fast and Sustained Weight Loss*:

> Following Atkin's recommendations could more than double your risk of certain cancers, especially meat-sensitive cancers, such as epithelial cancers of the respiratory tract...

> ...It is not only that his menu plans are incredibly high in saturated fat, it is that Atkins's menus prohibit and restrict the foods known to offer powerful protection against cancer.... fruit exclusion alone is a significant cancer marker."[8]

And while high-protein plans may help you lose weight initially, they won't help you keep it off long-term. That's because the only way you'll be able to keep the weight off is if you continue to restrict your carbohydrate intake, which includes healthy carbs like fresh fruits and vegetables, so that your body remains in ketosis.

Ketosis, a state in which the body produces increased levels of ketones, is the selling point of Atkins and other low carb plans. Ketosis occurs when the body begins burning mostly fat for fuel instead of carbohydrates.

By eating a low-carbohydrate diet like Atkins, you force your body into ketosis and lose body fat. While this may help you lose weight in the beginning, it will likely be very difficult to keep it off. As soon as you increase your carbohydrate intake—even if it's just fresh fruits and vegetables—you will no longer be in ketosis and you will gain weight.

Casein: A Scary Carcinogen?

Casein is not just the primary protein found in dairy. According to Dr. Campbell, it promotes cancer as well.

Campbell conducted an experiment in which he gave one group of rats aflatoxin (a toxin in mold linked to liver cancer) and a 20% protein diet and another group the same amount of aflatoxin but a diet containing only 5% protein.

After 100 weeks, the rats fed the 20% protein diet were "dead or near death from liver tumors," while the rats fed the 5% diet were "alive, active and thrifty, with sleek hair coats".[1]

In humans, a gluten-free, casein-free diet has been shown to be an affective treatment for autism, Asperger's, and other autism spectrum disorders.[89-90]

How Much Do We Really Need?

As it turns out, human protein needs are very small. All authorities do not agree on the specific amount, but as John Robbins writes in his revolutionary book *Diet for a New America: How Your Food Choices Affect Your Health, Happiness, and the Future of Life on Earth*:

...their calculations do fall within a specific range. It is a range that runs from a low estimate of two and a half percent of our total daily calories up to a high estimate of over eight percent. The figures at the high end include built-in safety margins, and are not 'minimum' allowances, but rather 'recommended' allowances."[139]

For instance, the Institute of Medicine recommends only 46 grams per day for women and 56 grams per day for men.[140] According to the Food and Agriculture Organization of the United Nations (FAO), only 7-8% of total calories need to come from protein.[141] On a 2,000 calorie diet, this amounts to 140-160 calories or a measly 35-40 grams of protein per day.

As I will show in chapter six, it's very easy to meet and even exceed these protein requirements on a raw vegan diet.

What a Vegan Diet Can Do For You

Did you know that a meat and egg-free diet can increase blood levels of dehydroepiandrosterone (DHEA), a hormone positively linked to female fertility and longevity, by as much as 20% in just 5 days?[142]

Did you know that a low-fat vegan diet can increase your metabolic rate, allowing you to burn more calories even when at rest?[143]

Did you know that a low-fat vegan diet has shown to be more effective at improving glycemic and lipid control in type II diabetics than a conventional diabetes diet?[144]

Did you know that a raw vegan diet full of fiber and antioxidants can reduce pain and joint stiffness in people with rheumatoid arthritis?[145]

Did you know that a study of over 69,000 participants found that vegans had a 16% decreased risk for developing cancer?[146]

Animal Products and Our Planet

We say that however close you can be to a vegan diet and further from the mean American diet, the better you are for the planet. ~ Gidon Eshel, Assistant Professor in Geophysical Sciences at the University of Chicago[147]

Eating a meat, milk, fish, and egg-rich diet isn't just detrimental to your health. The production and processing of such products is bad for the environment as well. Factory farming, in which large numbers of chickens, cows, pigs, or other farm animals are raised in confined living quarters, is one of the top environmental polluters.

According to a 2006 report by the Food and Agriculture Organization of the United Nations (FAO), energy production is the only process that emits more greenhouse gases than livestock production (chicken, pork, and beef).[148]

That's right. Eating animals is harder on the environment than driving your car, riding the bus, or taking the subway!

But that's not all.

Factory farming requires lots of land, water, and energy both for the livestock and for the livestock's food. This feed, mostly corn, is subjected to large amounts of pesticides, herbicides, and other contaminants that pollute our air, water, and soils. The animals themselves are pumped full of antibiotics, which also pollute the environment and lead to dangerous antibiotic-resistance microorganisms in our water, soil, and food supplies.

What about organic and grass-fed meats? Aren't these better for the environment?

Not necessarily. Studies have shown that organic milk production requires more land to produce, grass-fed cows emit more methane, and organic chicken is contaminated with harmful bacteria.[149, 150, 151]

Animal Products and Our Furry (and Scaly) Friends

"The vast majority of the animals we eat are not, as those in the animal agribusiness industry would have us believe, "contented cows" and "happy hens" lazing amid grassy fields and open barnyards...From the moment they are born, these animals are kept in intensive confinement where they may suffer from disease, exposure to extreme temperatures, severe overcrowding, violent handling, and even psychosis." ~ Melanie Joy, Ph.D., *Why We Love Dogs, Eat Pigs and Wear Cows: An Introduction to Carnism*

While everyone knows that the steak on their plate or the milk in their mug is the result of death and destruction, many don't know (or choose to ignore) the fact that the animals used to produce these foods suffer greatly long before the slaughter.

Below are just a few examples.

Beef cattle are fed a grain-based diet, which is cheap, fattening, and forces the cows to grow faster. Such an unnatural diet often results in painful bloat and liver abscesses.[153-155]

Dairy cows—besides being forced to live in stalls and produce several times more milk than they ever could naturally—are often subjected to tail banding, "in which a rubber band or similar ligature is wrapped tightly around the tail at the desired point of removal. This cuts off the blood supply to the end of the tail, which atrophies and usually falls away after a few days."[156]

Baby chicks have their beaks cut *without anesthesia* to avoid pecking and cannibalism, a direct result of their confined living quarters, in a painful process called "debeaking".[157]

Pigs are subjected to extreme weather conditions during transportation to slaughterhouses, during which many literally freeze to death or die of heat exhaustion.[152]

Wild fish captured by nets and bottom trawlers suffer decompression when brought on deck, resulting in "intense internal pressure" that "ruptures their swim bladders, pops out their eyes, and pushes their esophagi and stomachs out through their mouths."[158]

While animals raised in cruelty-free environments and slaughtered in the most humane ways possible are out there—although many "free-range" and "cage-free" animals are anything but—these animals still must be killed before they can be eaten.

As author Melanie Joy, ph.D. states in *Why We Love Dogs, Eat Pigs, and Wear Cows*:

> In much of the industrialized world, we eat meat not because we have to; we eat meat because we choose to. We don't need meat to survive or even to be healthy; millions of healthy and long-lived vegetarians have proven this point. We eat animals simply because it's what we've always done, and because we like the way they taste. Most of us eat animals because it's just the way things are.[152]

If you would like more information on the devastating effects of factory farming, check out *Why We Love Dogs, Eat Pigs, and Wear Cows* by Melanie Joy, *Eating Animals* by Safran Foer, and *Slaughterhouse* by Gail Eisnitz.

Vegan is Where It's At

If you want to avoid (and even reverse) 14 out of the top 15 leading causes of death—including heart disease, cancer, diabetes, Alzheimer's disease, liver disease, hypertension, Parkinson's disease, and even influenza and pneumonia—stop eating animal products.[159]

If you want to significantly reduce your carbon footprint, stop eating animal products.

If you want to help put an end to animal cruelty for ALL animals, stop eating animal products.

CHAPTER 2
Why Low-Fat?

One of the major selling points of a vegan diet is that it's a healthy way to eat. Just get rid of the meat and milk and voila!

Ah, if only things were that easy.

Unfortunately, giving up animal products is not the only requirement of a healthy diet. In fact, it's very easy to eat a very UNHEALTHY diet that's totally devoid of animal products.

Just take a look at this list of junk foods.

- **Charm's lollipops**
- **Cracker Jacks**
- **Fritos**
- **Lay's Potato Chips**
- **Nabisco Oreo Cookies**
- **Sour Patch Kids**
- **Mary Janes**
- **Krispy Kreme Fruit Pies**
- **Kool-Aid Gels**
- **Jolly Ranchers**
- **Fireballs**
- **Famous Amos Sandwich Cookies**
- **7-Eleven 7 Select Strawberry Creme Cookies**

It may be hard to believe, but all of these sugary, fatty, processed foods contain no animal products whatsoever.[1] You could literally live on french fries, potato chips, and soda and still be 100% vegan!

And of course, we can't forget about all of the processed food items that are marketed specifically for vegans. Products like soy hotdogs, bean burgers, and rice ice creams, just to name a few. These may be vegan, but they're still processed and often high in fat, full of sodium, and contain nerve-damaging ingredients like MSG.[2-3]

If your goal is to be healthy, you can't just give up meat and milk. You've got to take things a step further...

Rule #1: Cut Back on Fat

As I mentioned in the last chapter, eating lots of saturated fat is unwise. Saturated fat has been implicated in numerous health concerns, including cardiovascular disease, type II diabetes, breast cancer, prostate cancer, and colorectal cancer.

When you adopt a vegan diet, you automatically reduce your consumption of saturated fats because you avoid meat, milk, and other animal products which are high in this type of fat.

But going vegan doesn't mean that you're automatically reducing your *total* fat intake. In fact, it's very easy to consume way too much fat without *any* animal products in your diet.

For instance, if you're eating french fries, potato chips, breakfast cereals, or other vegan junk foods, you're consuming potentially large amounts of another not-so-healthy fat: trans fat. Found in large quantities in processed foods, trans fat has been linked to heart disease, diabetes, obesity and various cancers, as well as Alzheimer's Disease, depression, and even aggression.[4-7, 8-10, 11, 12-14, 15, 16, 17]

Okay, so you've already cut out the saturated AND processed trans fats. Job well done, right?

Not quite. It's possible—dare I say probable?—that you are still eating too much fat.

Plant Fat is Still Fat

Even if you avoid processed foods of any kind, there are still several fatty foods available to you on a vegan diet.

Avocados are one example. Over 75% of the calories in a Hass avocado come from fat. Nuts and seeds are high in fat as well, along with olives and mature coconut meat.

But if these foods are not high in saturated or trans fats, where does the fat come from?

The fat in these whole plant foods are of predominantly two types: monounsaturated and polyunsaturated. While these fats are not as harmful as saturated or trans fats, they do present numerous health concerns if consumed in high enough quantities.

Here are a few reasons why you may want to limit monounsaturated and polyunsaturated fats in your diet.

Plant Fats and Body Fat

One gram of carbohydrate or protein is 4 calories. One gram of fat is 9 calories. That's an additional 5 calories for every gram of fat you consume.

As a result, high-fat foods are high-calorie foods. Half of one Hass avocado (less than three ounces) is over 100 calories. One handful of almonds (about one ounce) is over 150 calories. Three ounces of coconut meat is just over 300 calories.

On the other hand, half of one banana is 50 calories, an ounce of blueberries is 16 calories, and three ounces of romaine is 15 calories.

The more fat you consume, the more calories you consume. If you consume more calories than your body needs, you will gain weight.

Even if you don't consume more calories than you need, the potential for weight gain is there simply because the human body is more efficient at storing dietary fat as body fat than it is at storing carbohydrates as body fat. In other words, you burn more calories converting carbohydrates to body fat than you do converting dietary fat to body fat.[18]

Plant Fats and Nutrient-Density

Nutrient-density refers to the ratio of nutrients to calories. A high nutrient-density is good because it means you will take in a lot of nutrients per calorie. Lower nutrient-density means you must eat more to get the nutrients you need. Eating more means more calories, and more calories means weight gain.

For the most part, fatty plant foods like avocados and nuts are less nutrient dense than vegetables, fruits, legumes, and whole grains.[19]

For instance, let's compare 100 calories of romaine to 100 calories of plain potato chips.

Table 2.1 Nutrient Comparison of Romaine Lettuce and Plain Potato Chips

Nutrients	Romaine Lettuce, raw (100 calories)	Potato Chips, plain, salted (100 calories)
Vitamin A	51235.3 IU	0
Folate	800 mcg	13.8 mcg
B1	0.4 mg	0
B2	0.4 mg	0
B3	1.8 mg	0.8 mg
B5	0.8 mg	0.8 mg
B6	0.4 mg	0.1 mg
Vitamin C	23.5 mg	3.4 mg
Vitamin E	0.8 mg	1.2 mg
Vitamin K	602.9 mcg	4.1 mcg
Calcium	194.1 mg	4.4 mg
Copper	0.3 mg	0.1 mg
Iron	5.7 mg	0.3 mg
Magnesium	82.4 mg	12.9 mg
Manganese	0.9 mg	0.1 mg
Phosphorus	176.5 mg	28.6 mg
Potassium	1452.9 mg	202 mg
Selenium	2.4 mcg	1.5 mg
Sodium	47.1 mg	88.6 mg
Zinc	1.4 mg	0.4 mg

Source: *http://cronometer.com/*

As you can see, the romaine contains far more nutrients than the potato chips, which are little more than empty calories and salt. No matter how many chips you eat, you'd never be able to acquire the nutrients found in just 100 measly calories of romaine.

Now let's compare 100 calories of romaine to 100 calories of pistachio nuts.

Table 2.2 Nutrient Comparison of Romaine Lettuce and Pistachio Nuts

Nutrients	Romaine Lettuce, raw (100 calories)	Pistachio Nuts, raw (100 calories)
Vitamin A	51235.3 IU	73.8 IU
Folate	800 mcg	9.1 mcg
B1	0.4 mg	0.2 mg
B2	0.4 mg	0
B3	1.8 mg	0.2 mg
B5	0.8 mg	0.1 mg
B6	0.4 mg	0.3 mg
Vitamin C	23.5 mg	1.0 mg
Vitamin E	0.8 mg	0.4 mg
Vitamin K	602.9 mcg	0 mcg
Calcium	194.1 mg	18.7 mg
Copper	0.3 mg	0.2 mg
Iron	5.7 mg	0.7 mg
Magnesium	82.4 mg	21.5 mg
Manganese	0.9 mg	0.2 mg
Phosphorus	176.5 mg	87.2 mg
Potassium	1452.9 mg	182.4 mg
Selenium	2.4 mcg	1.2 mcg
Sodium	47.1 mg	0.2 mg
Zinc	1.4 mg	0.4 mg

Source: http://cronometer.com/

Like the potato chips, the pistachio nuts can't compete with the romaine. You would have to eat far more nuts—which means more calories, more fat, and more fat on your body—to equal the amount of nutrients found in 100 calories of romaine.

Do Nuts Really Lower Your Cholesterol?

Based on the evidence, a serving or two of nuts eaten several times per week does seem to improve cholesterol levels, but the amount is verging on insignificant. A pooled analysis of 25 dietary intervention trials found that consuming 67 grams (2.4 ounces) of nuts per day reduced total cholesterol levels by 10.9 mg, a 5.1% change.[34]

So if you had a blood cholesterol level of 300 mg/dL, with below 150 mg/dL being ideal, eating 2.4 ounces of nuts each day would only reduce your cholesterol by a few points. At 289 mg/dL, your total cholesterol level would still be far too high.

And remember, nuts are high-calorie foods. Just 2.4 ounces of nuts is over 400 calories! Unless you were diligent about tracking your food intake, it would be very easy to overeat by including so many nuts in your diet.

Switching to a low fat, plant-based diet would be a much better choice for lowering cholesterol and improving heart health than increasing your nut consumption. It's not unheard of for participants of such plant-based plans, like Dr. John McDougall's and Dr. Joel Fuhrman's programs, to see drops in total cholesterol of 100 points or more.[35-36]

Plant Fats and the Omega-6 to Omega-3 Ratio

You've probably heard about the essential fatty acids omega-6 (linoleic acid) and omega-3 (alpha-linolenic acid) and their importance in a healthy diet. What you may not have heard about is the importance of the omega-6 to omega-3 ratio.

Many experts agree that the ideal ratio is 1:1 to 2:1 of omega 6 to omega 3 fatty acids, perhaps as much as 4:1.[20-23] While a few varieties of seeds like chia and flax contain a healthy omega-6 to omega-3 ratio, most fatty plant foods do not. Most contain far more omega-6 fatty acids than omega-3s.

Table 2.3 Omega-6:Omega-3 Ratio in Avocado, Nuts, & Seeds

Overt Fats*	Omega-6:Omega-3
Avocado, California	15:1
Almonds	2004:1
Brazil Nuts	1139:1
Cashew Nuts	125:1
Chia Seeds	1:3
English Walnuts	4:1
Flaxseed	1:4
Hazelnuts (filberts)	90:1
Macadamia Nuts	6:1
Pecans	21:1
Pine Nuts	300:1
Pistachios	52:1
Pumpkin Seeds	114:1
Sesame Seeds	57:1

Source: http://cronometer.com/

*Overt fats are foods predominated by fat. Hass avocados are overt because they contain roughly 77% fat. Other overt fats include nuts and seeds like walnuts and pumpkin seeds, olives, mature coconut meat, and oils.

All of this is important because a diet with an unhealthy ratio that's high in omega-6s and low in omega-3s—like the Standard American Diet that has a ratio above 10:1—is pro-inflammatory and has been tied to numerous diseases and disorders, including cardiovascular disease, obesity, chronic obstructive pulmonary disease (COPD), breast cancer, and prostate cancer.[20-21 & 24, 25-26, 27-28, 29, 30, 31]

In addition, high amounts of omega-6 fatty acids can actually replace and reduce omega-3 fats in the body, inhibiting the conversion of ALA (omega-3) to EPA and DHA. This is particularly concerning for vegans, who tend to consume a diet high in omega-6s, low in omega-3s, and completely devoid of EPA and DHA.[*32]

Plant Fats and Insulin Resistance

Insulin is a hormone produced by the pancreas that aids in blood glucose regulation. Following a meal, the concentration of glucose in your bloodstream increases. Your pancreas will then release insulin in order to carry the glucose out of your blood and into the cells of your liver, muscle, and adipose (fat) tissues.[37]

This is what happens in a normal, properly functioning body. In people who are insulin resistant, however:

> ...their muscle, fat, and liver cells do not respond properly to insulin. As a result, their bodies need more insulin to help glucose enter cells. The pancreas tries to keep up with this increased demand for insulin by producing more. Eventually, the pancreas fails to keep up with the body's need for insulin.[38]

This is what's known as insulin resistance, a risk factor for type II diabetes.[38]

One of the contributing factors of insulin resistance is fat intake. Saturated fat, linoleic acid (omega-6), and oleic acid (monounsaturated) have all been linked to insulin resistance.[39, 40]

Plant Fats and Metabolic Acidosis

Like meat and dairy, nuts and seeds are acid-forming. If eaten in large amounts, these foods can potentially lead to bone and muscle loss.

Plant Fats and Seasonality

If you were living like your hunter-gatherer ancestors, how many fatty plant foods do you think you would come across? Probably not many.

---

* EPA (eicosapentaenoic acid) and DHA (docosahexaenoic acid) are two long-chain omega-3 fatty acids. They are not essential because the human body can convert short-chain omega-3 fatty acids—like those found in walnuts and chia seeds, for example—to EPA and then to DHA, provided enough omega-3 is present in the diet. However, some people (particularly elderly vegan men) appear to have a hard time making the conversion and may require supplementation.23 & 33

You certainly wouldn't have bags of shelled pistachios or jars of tahini at your fingertips.

That's because the harvest season for nuts and seeds is pretty short, usually during the autumn months.

What About Oils?

You may have noticed that I haven't talked much about oils. There's a good reason for this. While whole foods like avocados, nuts, and seeds are indeed healthy, the oils that are produced from these foods are not.

Oils are junk foods no better than granulated sugar. In my opinion, they're actually worse!

First, oil contains more calories than sugar. Just one tablespoon of coconut oil is almost 120 calories while the same amount of sugar is less than half of that.

Second, oil is 100% fat. Some oils also contain small amounts of vitamins E and K, but for the most part they're just fat and a good bit of this fat is saturated.

In fact, did you know that just two tablespoons of olive oil contains over seven times the amount of saturated fat found in three ounces of skinless chicken breast? Two tablespoons of coconut oil contains even more—47 times more!

Third, most oils have a very poor omega-6 to omega -3 fatty acid ratio. Olive oil is 11:1, sunflower oil is 15:1, and corn oil is a whopping 79:1!

Fourth, oils are prone to oxidation which causes rancidity and the production of free radicals. Free radicals are unstable molecules that have been linked to aging, cardiovascular disease, and even cancer.[41]

But what about olive oil? It's supposed to be super heart-healthy, right?

One study found that all fats—including oleic acid, the predominating fat in olive oil— "significantly increased risk" of new arterial lesions in subjects with coronary heart disease.[42]

Another study found that several oils, including olive oil, are as bad as butter when it comes to blood clotting![43]

Not so heart-healthy after all.

One of the best things you can do for your health, including your heart, is to cut out oils completely. Just by removing two tablespoons of olive oil from your daily diet, you'll save over 230 calories and 27 grams of fat every day.

How Much Fat Do We Really Need?

Like protein, we need very little fat in our diets. And while not everyone agrees on the exact percentage, most plant-based diet experts agree that fatty foods should be limited and recommend less than 10% or no more than 10% of total calories from fat.[*] [**44-50]

On a 2,000 calorie diet of whole plant foods, 10% works out to around one ounce of nuts or seeds per day, 1/2 an avocado, or 2 ounces of mature coconut meat per day.

Final Word on Fats

Plant fats like nuts and avocados are healthy foods, but fats of all kinds should be kept to a minimum. Oils, including "heart-healthy" olive oil, are nothing but empty calories and should be avoided completely.[***]

Rule #2: Fill Up on Carbs

So now we know that humans need very small amounts of protein and fat in their diets, about 20% or less of total calories. On a 2,000 calorie diet, that works out to less than 400 calories coming from protein AND fat per day.

What about the remaining 80%? The answer is carbohydrates.

---

[*]   Fat comes from whole, plant-based sources and generally does not include any oils.

[**]   Dr. Joel Fuhrman recommends that 10-40% of total calories come from avocados, nuts, and seeds.[51]

[***] Wondering how to make a tasty salad dressing without oil? Use whole fats instead! Just a little bit of blended avocado or soaked nuts/seeds will make for an incredibly rich and creamy dressing. Here's a favorite recipe of mine: 1 ounce raw pistachios, juice from one lemon, celery powder and cumin to taste, and water. Blend and pour over your favorite greens. Delicious!

I know, I know. You've been told for years how bad carbs are for you, how they're nothing but empty calories that make you tired, sick, and flabby.

This is true *if* we're talking about refined carbohydrates.

There are two types of carbohydrates: whole and refined. Your whole carbs include foods like fruits, vegetables, legumes, and whole grains like brown rice, oats and whole wheat. Refined carbs include processed foods like breads, cakes, cookies, chips, and pastas.

It's the latter that gets the bad rap and for good reason. Whole carbohydrates are full of nutrients and low in fat. Refined carbohydrates have had many of their nutrients destroyed via processing and are often combined with lots of fat, salt, and unhealthy food additives like artificial sweeteners and MSG.

Below I've compared a whole carbohydrate (brown rice) to a refined carbohydrate (white rice).

Table 2.4 Nutrient Comparison of Brown Rice and White Rice

Nutrients	Brown rice, raw (100 calories)	White rice, raw, unenriched (100 calories)
Vitamin A	0 IU	0 IU
Folate	5.5 mcg	2.5 mcg
Thiamin	0.1 mg	<0.1 mg
Riboflavin	<0.1 mg	<0.1 mg
Niacin	1.2 mg	0.4 mg
Pantothenic Acid	0.4 mg	0.4 mg
Pyridoxine	0.1 mg	<0.1 mg
Vitamin C	0 mg	0 mg
Vitamin E	0 mg	0 mg
Vitamin K	0 mcg	0 mcg
Calcium	9.1 mg	2.5 mg

Nutrients	Brown rice, raw (100 calories)	White rice, raw, unenriched (100 calories)
Copper	0.1 mg	<0.1 mg
Iron	0.5 mg	0.2 mg
Magnesium	39.5 mg	9.7 mg
Manganese	1.0 mg	0.3 mg
Phosphorus	72.9 mg	30 mg
Potassium	74 mg	23.9 mg
Selenium	0 mcg	0 mg
Sodium	1.1 mg	0.3 mg
Zinc	0.6 mg	0.3 mg

Source: http://cronometer.com/

The brown rice contains more nutrients than the white in almost every single category. This should come as no surprise since white rice is simply brown rice with the germ and bran removed.

Carbs and Nutrient-Density

The most nutrient-dense foods on the planet—those foods that contain the most nutrients per calorie—are vegetables (particularly green vegetables), legumes, fruits, and whole grains.[19] All of these foods are whole carbohydrates.

On the other hand, the least nutrient dense foods are refined sugars, refined oils, refined grains, meat, dairy, and eggs. None of these are whole, unprocessed carbohydrates.

Carbs and Your Sweet Tooth

Let's face it. Dinner isn't complete without a big bowl of ice cream or a gargantuan piece of pie to seal the deal.

According to biologist Jason Cryan, there's some logic behind our love of the sweet stuff:

...we have physiologically associated a sweet taste with high-energy foods which would have helped our earliest ancestors survive better in their environment...When one considers our ability to taste, our ability to perceive 'sweet' is relatively weak, while our ability to perceive 'bitter' is generally considered much stronger...evolving a low tolerance to 'bitter' and a high tolerance to 'sweet' might have promoted our ancestors to actively seek out sweet tasting foods.[52]

In other words, we have a sweet tooth for a reason. Our species has evolved to seek out sweet foods like fresh fruit so that is the taste our tongues are most sensitive too.

Carbs and Energy

Glucose is the primary energy source for every cell in the human body. Glucose is a simple sugar (i.e. a carbohydrate) found in fruits vegetables, grains, and legumes.*

Carbs and Satiation

Several studies have shown that carbohydrates are more satiating—in some cases *significantly* so—than fats.[53-55] While high-fat meals leave you hungry and craving more fatty foods, high-carbohydrate meals leave you satisfied and wanting less food at your next meal.**

Focus on Whole Foods

Remember that when I say "carbs," I'm not talking about potato chips, pastries, or pastas. I'm talking about unprocessed foods like fresh fruits and vegetables.

I'm also not talking about the so-called healthy products marketed towards vegans. As I mentioned earlier in this chapter, these products are not much different from your regular junk foods. They're highly processed, high in calories, and are often full of fat and unwanted additives.

---

* Yes, glucose is sugar. Don't be alarmed! There is a huge difference between refined sugary foods like candy and whole sugary foods like fruit. For much more information on sugar and fruit, please see chapter five.

** It's also important to note that these high-carbohydrate meals are usually high in fiber as well. High-carbohydrate meals that are low in fiber (i.e. refined carbohydrates) are not as satiating.[53 & 56]

How Much is Too Much?

Unlike protein and fat, eating "too many carbs" is virtually impossible.

For one, there's no issue with eating a diet high in carbohydrates like there is with one high in protein/fat...assuming you aren't eating too many calories overall or loading up on refined carbs, of course.

Plus, it's much more difficult to overeat carbohydrates, particularly fresh fruits and vegetables, because they are lower in calories and more satiating.

Final Word on Carbs

Carbohydrates are the foundation of a healthy diet. They're high in nutrients, low in calories, satiating, and delicious.

Putting It All Together

The ideal human diet is one that is both low in fat and high in carbohydrates. Limit your total fat intake to around 10% and eat all the whole carbohydrates you like.[*]

What about protein?

As I mentioned in the first chapter, our protein needs are very small. You'll meet your protein needs on virtually any diet as long as you consume enough calories.[**]

---

[*]   Ideally, I recommend avoiding grains and legumes all together, or at least limiting them. For all the reasons why, please see chapter four.

[**]   For more on getting enough protein on a raw vegan diet, please see chapter six.

CHAPTER 3
Why Raw?

I've shown you why you should stop eating animal products. I've shown you why you should cut back on the fat and load up on the carbohydrates.

In this third chapter, I'll show you why you should take one final step and go raw. But before I do that, I need to dispel a few myths that have been giving the raw food movement a bad name for far too long.

The Wrong Reasons to Eat Raw

Raw Myth #1: All Wild Animals Eat Raw So We Should Too

Yes, all wild animals eat a raw food diet. So what?

No other species cooks its food because no other species *can* cook its food, just like no other species can read, write, or stay up until 3am playing Words With Friends on their iPhones.

More importantly, the fact that no creatures living in the wild cook their foods doesn't tell us anything about eating raw, such as which raw foods to eat and how much. It also doesn't tell us anything about cooking itself, like whether or not cooking our foods is actually harmful.

Raw Myth #2: Humans Have Not Adapted to Eating Cooked Foods

Actually, there *have* been small adaptations in human physiology as a result of eating cooked food.

Malocclusion, or misalignment of the teeth, is one example. Experts believe this malformation is largely a result of eating soft cooked foods, which doesn't require as much work from our jaw muscles as fibrous raw foods.[1-3] more evidence?

An increase in amylase production is another likely adaptation to cooked foods. Amylase is a salivary enzyme needed to produce starch. More of this enzyme suggests a higher intake of starchy foods like potatoes and cereal grains, which is exactly what has happened since the advent of cooking.[4-5]

Finally, our digestive tract is smaller, which is also likely a result of cooking.[6-7]

→ enough not evidence?

Raw Myth #3: Cooking is EVIL!

You may be laughing, but this belief is not uncommon within the raw food world. Some raw foodists honestly believe that cooking foods is "wrong" and see the advent of using fire to heat food as an "evil" discovery.

With the abundance and variety of fresh fruits and vegetables available today, we don't need to rely on high-calorie cooked foods to meet our nutritional needs. But of course, this wasn't always the case.

For a portion of human existence, cooked foods were absolutely vital. Cooking made foods like meat and starchy grains, legumes, and tubers easier to digest. And according to primatologist Richard Wrangham, this fact meant that less energy was required for digestion, which meant more could be used for brain growth.[7]

In other words, it may very well have been cooked foods that made us human.[7]

Raw Myth #4: Raw Food is Living Food

You've probably heard raw food described as "living" food and the enzymes in raw foods as "alive."

Certainly a head of romaine lettuce growing in the ground is alive. But what about when that romaine is harvested, packaged, shipped to a warehouse, and finally shelved in a store. Is the romaine still alive?

And what about when you chop, slice, blend, juice, dehydrate and chew the romaine? Is it alive then?

Of course not.

And as far as enzymes are concerned, saying enzymes are "alive" is like saying carbohydrates or fat or protein is "alive". Enzymes are just catalysts (most are proteins), which are neither alive nor dead.

Speaking of enzymes...

Raw Myth #5: Cooking Kills Plant Enzymes that are Necessary for Optimal Digestion and Good Health

Possibly the most cited reason for eating raw is because cooking food destroys the food's enzymes. While it's true that most food enzymes are damaged at low temperatures (around 115 degrees), is this really such a big deal?

According to most raw foodists, yes, because the enzymes present in raw foods actually assist in your body's digestion of those foods. When you heat a food and destroy its enzymes, you force your body to produce more of its own enzymes to properly digest that food when you eat it.[8]

This is a big concern because supposedly we can only produce a limited amount of digestive enzymes during our lifetime. If we cook our food, we are using up more of these precious enzymes, which could lead to an enzyme deficiency and poor health as we age.[9]

41

These theories—that food enzymes are necessary for human health and that our capacity to produce digestive enzymes is limited—stem from Dr. Edward Howell's 1985 book *Enzyme Nutrition: The Food Enzyme Concept*.[10]

Enzyme Deficiency Causes Disease

As evidence that enzyme deficiency causes disease, Dr. Howell turns to nature. Unlike modern-day humans, Howell explains, wild animals are "healthy" and "disease-free." Vitamin and mineral sufficiency cannot explain their good health because human foods have been "fortified to the hilt" and yet we are a disease-ridden species. The only answer is "superb enzyme nutrition" that results from eating raw foods.[10]

First, wild animals are most certainly not "healthy" and "disease-free". Along with infectious diseases like Lyme disease and rabies, wild animals do suffer from chronic degenerative diseases like oral diseases and osteoarthritis despite their all-raw diets.*[11-12]

Second, regardless of fortification, many people today are nutrient-deficient. Deficiencies of vitamin C, vitamin D, vitamin B6, vitamin B12, and iron are common amongst people in the United States and can cause various serious illnesses including anemia, osteomalacia (rickets), and irreversible nerve damage.[13, 14, 15, 16, 17, 18, 19]

And as I showed in chapter one of this book, many people today tend to consume too many overall calories, fat, cholesterol, protein, and preformed vitamin A, a dietary pattern that has been positively linked to heart disease, diabetes, osteoporosis, and cancer.

But let's say that Howell is right. Let's say that malnutrition has nothing to do with the current state of human health. Does that prove that the diseases and disorders that plague us are caused by an enzymatic deficiency?

Of course not. The only thing it proves is that malnutrition *doesn't* cause human disease. It says nothing about what actually *does* cause disease.

---

* Although the rates of degenerative disease in wild animals are typically much lower than what we find in zoo animals and humans living in industrialized nations.

To prove that enzyme deficiency is what causes disease, we need evidence. Howell's mere speculation that enzyme abundance is why wild animals lead healthier lives is not evidence.

Enzyme Production is Limited

As evidence that the human body produces a finite number of digestive enzymes, what Howell calls the "enzyme potential," he turns to studies showing that older individuals produce less enzymes than younger ones. According to Howell, researchers found that "the enzyme of the saliva in young adults was 30 times stronger than in persons over 69 years old."[10]

Whether or not this research actually proves that we produce less enzymes as we age—the book includes no formatted list of references—is irrelevant to Howell's claim that the human body has a fixed number of enzymes it can produce.

As enzyme researcher Stephen Rothman puts it, "a decrease in the rate of secretion over time and some sort of timed 'finite limit' are quite different things. There is no finite limit on what we produce; we continue to do so as long as we are alive."[20]

Enzyme Nutrition: Science or Science Fiction?

Howell continues on this course, making grandiose claims with little to no evidence to back up his theories, for the rest of the book. The works that are cited—again, there is no list of references—are completely out-of-date, with most research published pre-1950 even though *Enzyme Nutrition* was published in 1985.[10]

Not that there is an abundance of current-day research proving Howell's theories. There is some evidence that certain plant enzymes may assist in our own digestion and may even help prevent cancer, but that's about it.

I'll talk more about enzyme research later in the chapter. For now, let's look at some more raw myths.

Raw Myth #6: Cooking Denatures Protein and Renders it Useless to the Body

The myth here is not with the statement that cooking denatures protein, which it does. The issue is whether or not cooking protein actually renders it useless.

When something is denatured, its biological structure is changed. In the case of protein, denaturation destroys the secondary and tertiary structures, but leaves the primary structure (the amino acids) intact.*

Cooking isn't the only way to denature proteins. Your own body denatures the food you eat as a way to break down the protein and absorb the oh-so important amino acids.

Now for the big question: Is protein denaturation that's caused by cooking the same as protein denaturation that happens naturally as part of human digestion?

If it's not and cooking actually renders protein useless, then we would expect to see a lower absorption rate. In other words, we would expect our bodies to absorb less of the protein from food that is cooked than from the same food in its raw state.

Instead, it's well known that conservative cooking IMPROVES protein bioavailability in certain foods.** For example, cooking beans makes the protein more digestible because it inactivates anti-nutrients that would otherwise inhibit absorption.[22]

In any event, have you ever actually met anyone with a protein deficiency? If raw foodists were right and cooking really renders protein useless, then wouldn't everyone eating a diet predominated by cooked foods (aka virtually every person on the planet) have a protein deficiency?

---

* This denatured or "unfolded" state is sometimes reversible.[21]

** Conservative cooking refers to cooking foods at lower temperatures (e.g. steaming and boiling) for short durations.

Raw Myth #7: Eating Cooked Food Causes Digestive Leukocytosis

Digestive leukocytosis is a condition in which the white blood cell (WBC) count in your body rises after a meal. This is a potential concern because your white blood cells' job is to destroy unwanted materials, like pathogens and toxins, in your body. So eating a meal that increases your WBC count suggests that there is something in the food that requires fending off.

In 1930, researcher Paul Kouchakoff reported that digestive leukocytosis only occurred after subjects consumed cooked foods.[23] Raw foodists have gone on to use this research as proof that a 100% raw food diet is necessary for good health.

Kouchakoff's findings are certainly interesting (albeit dated), but do they actually support eating an all-raw diet?

Not at all. According to Kouchakoff himself:

It has been proved possible to take, without changing the blood formula, every

> **kind of foodstuff which is habitually eaten now, but only by following this rule, viz: - that it must be taken along with raw products, according to a definite formula.**[23]

In other words, digestive leukocytosis can be avoided simply by adding some raw foods to a cooked meal. Kouchakoff did not advocate a completely raw food diet.

The Real Reasons to Eat Raw

Now that the many myths have been shattered, it's time to show off the real reasons to adopt a raw food diet.

Raw Reason #1: Raw is More Nutritious

Fruits and vegetables, particularly dark leafy greens, are extremely nutrient dense, meaning they're low in calories yet high in necessary nutrients like vitamin A, vitamin C, folate, calcium, iron, and zinc.

When you heat these foods (or any food, for that matter), some nutrients will be destroyed. The amount of nutrient loss depends upon several factors, including temperature and duration.

In other words, foods that are cooked at high temperatures and for long periods of time will suffer more nutrient damage than foods that are cooked at low temperatures for short periods of time.

Cooking and Vitamin Loss

According to the USDA (see Table 3.1 below), plant foods typically lose small to moderate amounts of their vitamins when cooked at mild temperatures.

Table 3.1 Percentage of Vitamin Loss in Boiled Plant Foods

Food	Percentage of Vitamin Loss When Boiled and Drained*
Greens	5-45%
Root Vegetables	10-35%
Other Vegetables	10-35%
Tomatoes	5-30%
Potatoes	5-20%
Sweet Potatoes	5-25%

Food	Percentage of Vitamin Loss When Boiled and Drained*
Nuts	5-20%
Legumes	15-40%**
Rice	5-40%
Oatmeal	10-30%

Source: USDA Table of Nutrient Retention Factors, Release 6 (2007)

Note: The amount lost depends upon the vitamin. For example, greens lose almost 50% of total vitamin C when boiled, but only 5% of vitamin A.

*Retention rate is slightly higher if the cooking water is used instead of drained.

**This range is for legumes cooked for 15-20 minutes. Legumes cooked for 45-75 minutes lose slightly more vitamins (15-55%), while legumes cooked for 2-2.5 hours lose substantially more (15-70%).

Of course, these are just averages. Nutrient loss will vary from food to food and from nutrient to nutrient, since some vitamins like vitamin C and folate are more sensitive to heat than others.

Phytochemicals

Most phytochemicals, or cancer-fighting compounds found in plants, are quite sensitive to heat. For instance, one study found that both boiling and steaming almost completely destroyed all of the sulforaphane present in raw broccoli.[24]

Another study found that while boiling increased the carotenoids in broccoli and the polyphenols in Brussels sprouts, it reduced almost all other phytochemicals in both fresh and frozen samples.[25]

And cruciferous vegetables like broccoli and Brussel sprouts aren't the only phytochemical-rich foods affected by heat. Research has shown that antioxidant content is significantly reduced when leafy greens are cooked.[26]

Vitamin C

It's well-known that vitamin C is very sensitive to heat, light, and oxygen. One study found that when green and purple-sprouting broccoli were boiled for 5 minutes, both varieties lost significant amounts of vitamin C (61.94% and 52.8%, respectively).[27]

Folate

Folate (vitamin B9), found in high amounts in leafy greens, is also very sensitive to heat. One study found that spinach retained only 49% of its folate while broccoli retained only 44%.[28*]

Doesn't cooking improve nutrient absorption?

It is true that certain nutrients like beta-carotene and lycopene are made more absorbable when heated. In fact, one study found that when eight females ate pureed carrots and spinach for four weeks, their plasma beta-carotene levels were *three times higher* than when they ate raw carrots and spinach, even though they were consuming the same amount of beta-carotene (9.3 mg/day) for both four-week periods![29]

However, it's important to note that in order to take in 9.3 mg of beta-carotene, the subjects had to consume 113 grams of each of the pureed carrots and spinach versus just 54.9 g of raw carrots and 39 g of raw spinach. They had to consume *more* of the vegetables when they are cooked than when they were raw.

This is significant because, as researchers Lilli B. Link and John D. Potter note in their review concerning vegetables and cancer risk, "although bioavailability is improved by cooking, if one ate equal quantities of these vegetables, raw and cooked, the plasma concentration of total and cis-β -carotene would likely be similar, and the α-carotene level would likely be higher by eating the raw vegetables."[30]

In other words, both raw and cooked vegetables are good sources of beta-carotene; raw because they contain more beta-carotene by weight and cooked because the beta-carotene is better absorbed. As I'll show you in chapter six, you'll take in TONS of beta-carotene and other carotenoids on a raw fruit and vegetable diet.

It's also important to remember that nutrition isn't limited to the 26 essential vitamins and minerals familiar to us all. There are thousands of other nutrients, some yet to be discovered, present in the fruits and vegetables we eat.

---

* However, the researchers found that both foods retain most of their folate when steamed.[28]

Take phytochemicals as an example. We did not even know that these cancer-fighting compounds existed until very recently. Today, scientists have discovered thousands of different phytochemicals and it's unknown how many more exist in our plant foods.

The fact that we haven't discovered all of the nutrients in our foods is particularly important with regards to phytochemicals since the majority of these compounds are sensitive to even relatively low levels of heat.

Cooking and Mineral Loss

Contrary to popular belief amongst raw foodies, most foods suffer very little to no mineral loss when boiled or steamed (see Table 3.2 below).

Table 3.2 Percentage of Mineral Loss in Boiled Plant Foods

Food	Percentage of Mineral Loss When Boiled and Drained*
Greens	5-15%**
Root Vegetables	5-10%
Other Vegetables	5-10%
Tomatoes	0%
Potatoes	5-10%
Sweet Potatoes	5-10%
Nuts	0%
Legumes	10-25%**
Rice	5-15%
Oatmeal	10-30%

Source: USDA Table of Nutrient Retention Factors, Release 6 (2007)

Note: The amount lost depends upon the mineral. For example, greens lose 15% of potassium when boiled, but only 5% of zinc.

*Retention rate is slightly higher if the cooking water is used instead of drained.

**This range is for legumes cooked for 15-20 minutes. Legumes cooked for 45-75 minutes and 2-2.5 hours lose slightly more minerals (10-35% and 10-45%, respectively).

So when it comes to minerals, there doesn't appear to be any advantage to consuming our foods raw versus steaming or boiling them.

Do Minerals Become Inorganic When Cooked?

Just like the belief that protein becomes unusable when cooked, the statement that the minerals in food revert to an inorganic state when heated is utter nonsense. Cooking may reduce the amount of certain minerals to some degree, but it cannot make them inorganic.

If you want proof, just look around you. It's well known that people who eat a standard processed, meaty Western diet consume way too much sodium and phosphorus. If cooking rendered these nutrients inorganic and therefore unusable by the body, wouldn't Americans be deficient in these as well as all other minerals?

Amino Acid Loss

Remember when I said that cooking denatures protein, but that this isn't a big deal because the primary structure (the amino acids) are left intact? Well, this isn't always the case.

It's well known that high-temperature cooking destroys essential amino acids, but more conservative cooking methods can as well.[31]

For instance, when flageolet beans were boiled for 32 or 37 minutes, "the content of all the amino acids fell," but only slightly. The one exception was tyrosine, which decreased from 35-45%.[32]

The essential amino acid lysine is particularly sensitive to heat, with one study showing that availability was "significantly depressed" when heated at 100°C (212°F) for just 15 minutes.[33] In another study, lysine was reduced by 13.2% and cysteine by 15% when chickpea seeds were cooked at 120°C (248°F) for 50 minutes.[34]

A study on bamboo shoots found that boiling for 10 minutes reduced all essential amino acids by approximately 20-56%.[*] Steaming, on the other hand, produced no significant reductions and actually increased the amount of the essential amino acid isoleucine by almost 4%.[35]

Enzyme Loss

Food enzymes are very heat-sensitive. Irreversible damage usually occurs at around 45°C (113°F) so even foods that are steamed for short durations no longer have their enzymes intact.

---

[*] Excluding threonine, which wasn't detected.[35]

50

As I explained earlier in this chapter, there's a lot of misinformation out there regarding plant enzymes and their effect on our own digestion and overall health. While many within the raw food world believe that enzymes are vitally important for human health, the evidence for this belief is sorely lacking.

That's why for years I believed that food enzymes played absolutely no role in our digestion or overall health. Here's a quote from an article I wrote in the spring of 2011 called "Is Apple Cider Vinegar Healthy?"

> **The idea that plant enzymes somehow help you digest your food is a huge misconception. The only enzymes that can function in your digestive system are your own digestive enzymes.**[36]

Then a raw reader turned me on to the book *Becoming Raw: The Essential Guide to Raw Vegan Diets* by Brenda Davis, RD and Vesanto Melina, MS, RD, in which I learned that food enzymes likely do a play a role—albeit a small one—in our digestion and overall health.[20]

Enzymes and Digestion

In terms of digestion, it's often assumed that food enzymes have no impact because they are destroyed by the gastric acid in the stomach. But as Davis and Melina point out, while food is stationed in the upper (proximal) portion of the stomach, the pH of the gastric acid ranges from 4.5 and 5.8. Since most food enzymes are denatured at a pH of less than 3.1, "we can expect that the enzymes naturally present in raw food would survive and be active during this time."*[20]

Again, the role here would be small. Once the enzymes pass the proximal stomach into the more acidic lower (distal) stomach, they are very likely completely denatured.

Enzymes and Cancer

In terms of health, there are two enzymes present in some plants that assist in our body's conversion of certain compounds to anti-carcinogenic phytochemicals. These enzymes are:

---

* The lower the pH, the more acidic the solution. So a pH of 1 is more acidic than a pH of 3 (100 times more) and a pH of 4 less so (100 times less).

1) myrosinase found in cruciferous vegetables like broccoli, cauliflower, cabbage, and kale, and
2) alliinase found in allium vegetables like garlic, onions, leeks, and chives.

Your body uses myrosinase to convert the glucosinolates in cruciferous vegetables to isothiocyanates, which are "highly prized for their ability to induce a group of enzymes in the body that help to inhibit cancer growth and kill cancer cells". [20] Your body uses alliinase to convert alliin in allium vegetables to allicin, a compound well-known for its anti-bacterial, anti-fungal, anti-arthritic, and anti-carcinogenic properties. [20]

Like most enzymes, myrosinase and alliinase are damaged at low temperatures, temperatures well below those used in conservative cooking methods like steaming and boiling. [20]

Final Word on Enzymes

So it seems that the enzymes found in plant foods actually do play a role in human digestion and health. While two enzymes present in two types of plants isn't exactly mind-blowing, Davis and Melina do note that not much research on food enzymes and human health has been conducted.

Hopefully this will change in the coming years.

Cooking and Fiber

While cooking doesn't destroy the fiber in fruits and vegetables, it can alter it. One study found that cooking vegetables increases the amount of soluble fiber while also reducing the amount of insoluble fiber.[37] Insoluble fiber binds to carcinogens, which helps in their elimination from the body.[38-39]

All or Mostly Raw?

A big debate today within the raw food movement is whether eating 100% raw foods is necessary for optimal health or if a mostly raw food diet that contains small amounts of cooked plant foods is just as healthy (if not better than) an all-raw diet.

First, a mostly raw food diet is an incredibly healthy diet.* ** Yes, the cooking process will destroy some nutrients and create some toxins, but the amount is very small.

Second, an all-raw diet isn't for everyone.

While I thoroughly enjoy feasting on fresh fruit, have no trouble getting in enough calories, love my super greens-filled salads, and don't struggle with cravings for cooked foods...I don't eat 100% raw. I use ingredients like roasted cacao powder (makes for a really delicious "hot chocolate" when blended with dates and warm water) and will eat things like rice paper (as part of a fresh spring wrap) on ocassion.

But that's just me. You may find that eating all-raw all the time works perfectly for you. Or you may find that eating all raw is just too difficult and sometimes not as satisfying as eating mostly raw with some cooked foods present in your diet.

Perhaps you continually struggle to get in enough calories eating 100% raw and find that cooked plant foods like rice and potatoes help you to feel satiated and maintain a healthy body weight. Perhaps you struggle to get in enough greens and other vegetables, foods that are absolutely vital for optimal health and well-being, and find that gently cooking these foods makes them more palatable so that you can eat more of them.

Maybe you live in a location that has subpar quality/variety of fresh fruit and vegetables during certain times of the year, making eating all-raw all the time virtually impossible. Maybe eating 100% raw foods puts a strain on your relationships with others while eating some cooked foods makes for more pleasant shared meal times.

---

* To be clear, a mostly raw diet is just that: a diet that's compromised of *mostly* raw, fresh foods. Here's a very simple example: a green smoothie for breakfast, bananas for lunch, and a huge salad followed by steamed potatoes and green beans with fresh salsa for dinner. And by cooked foods, I mean plant foods like vegetables, legumes, and grains that are heated for short durations at low temperatures (e.g. steaming and boiling).

** I didn't always feel this way. Like many, I used to believe that a 100% raw food diet was the only truly healthy diet. The evidence, not to mention the individual experiences of countless raw foodists, does not support this viewpoint.

Whatever the reason, there's no need to feel guilty or that your shortchanging yourself because you eat some cooked foods. As long as you are keeping your fat intake low and your carbohydrate intake high, while also filling up on whole plant foods and keeping processed foods to a minimum, you are doing your body a world of good.[*]

Raw Reason #2: Raw is Less Toxic

In chapter one, I talked a little bit about carcinogens like heterocyclic amines (HCAs) that form when food is cooked at high temperatures. While these dangerous chemicals are only produced in animal products like meat and eggs, there are other unwanted byproducts that form when plant foods are cooked.

Polycyclic Aromatic Hydrocarbons

Polycyclic aromatic hydrocarbons (PAHs) are carcinogenic chemicals formed in grilled, barbecued, and smoked meats. While plant foods like grains tend to be low in PAHs, cooking and refining these foods (e.g. breakfast cereals and pastries) can increase the amount they contain.[**][20 & 40]

The Maillard Reaction

The Maillard reaction is a form of non-enzymatic browning that occurs when high temperatures (around 300°F) are applied to certain foods. The browning of various items when cooked such as bread, sweet potatoes, carrots, tomatoes, legumes, and fruits is due to the Maillard reaction.

Not only can this process result in significant nutrient loss, it also creates harmful by-products such as advanced glycation end-products (AGEs) and acrylamide.[42, 43]

---

[*]   If you decide to include some cooked foods in your diet, I recommend keeping grains and legumes to a minimum due to their high anti-nutrient content. Vegetables like greens, broccoli, potatoes, and squashes are better choices. Stay tuned for more information on the many problems associated with the consumption of grains and legumes.

[**]   The amount of PAHs in a food will depend upon the amount in the soil. The more PAH in the soil, the more in the plant.[41]

Acrylamide

In 2002, it was discovered that when carbohydrates are cooked at high temperatures, acrylamide (a chemical used in water treatment) is formed.[44] Foods like bread, french fries, and potato chips contain large amounts of acrylamide, well above the limit that the World Health Organization (WHO) has set for drinking water.[44-45]

What's the big deal?

The big deal is that several animal studies have linked acrylamide consumption to various cancers, including kidney, breast, and ovarian cancers.[46] Human studies have also linked acrylamide consumption to certain cancers, including breast, ovarian, prostate, and bladder cancer.[46]

Most sources assert that acrylamide is not formed when food is boiled or steamed.45 However, in a 2005 joint meeting on food additives held by WHO and the Food and Agriculture Organization of the United Nations, it was agreed that, "although trace amounts of acrylamide can be formed by boiling, significant formation generally requires a processing temperature of 120°C [248°F] or higher."[44]

For instance, one study found acrylamide in boiled baking potatoes. Yes, the amount was small (less than 30 mcg/kg), but acrylamide was found.[47] Another study analyzing various popular foods on the Italian market showed small amounts of acrylamide (less than 50 mcg/kg) in rice that had been boiled for ten minutes.[48]

As the World Health Organization states on their website:

> **Acrylamide belongs to the group of chemicals thought to have no reliably identifiable 'threshold' of effects, meaning that very low concentrations will also result in very low risks, but not in zero risk: some risk is always present when the chemical is ingested.[45]**

This is why both the EPA and WHO have set the limit of acrylamide in drinking water to just 0.5 micrograms per liter (approximately 0.12

mcg per 8 ounces). The European Union has an even lower limit of 0.1 mcg/L of water.[45]

When it comes to acrylamide, we simply need more sensitive tests and more research, particularly on acrylamide levels in boiled and steamed non-tuberous vegetables. When it comes to my health, I choose to play it safe. I'll stick to the foods which I know contain the most nutrients and the least toxins: fresh fruits and vegetables.

Nuts and Seeds: Raw or Roasted?

Roasting nuts and seeds can lead to lipid oxidation, which causes the oils to go rancid.[49] Rancid fat is carcinogenic and pro-inflammatory.[50]

Roasting nuts and seeds can form trans fatty acids.[49]

Roasting nuts and seeds high in asparagine such as almonds can form significant amounts of acrylamide.[51]

Roasting nuts and seeds can form carboxymethyllysine, an advanced glycation end-product (AGE).[49] AGEs have been linked to cardiovascular and Alzheimer's diseases.[52, 53]

When it comes to nuts and seeds, raw is the best choice.

Raw Reason #3: Raw is Full of Water

While we can easily live for several weeks without any food, we can't last more than a few days without water. Even mild dehydration can cause fatigue, headaches, dizziness, constipation, and dry skin.[54]

That's because every one of your bodily processes requires water for proper functioning. And unlike your standard dehydrating processed diets that require you to drink 8-12 glasses of water everyday, fresh fruits and vegetables are full of this necessary nutrient. Even seemingly dry bananas are 75% water!

Raw Reason #4: Raw is Full of Fiber

Just like water, fiber is absolutely essential for good health. It makes for good digestion, keeps you feeling fuller for longer after your meals, and even helps in the elimination of toxins from your body!

And what foods are best for increasing your fiber intake? Fresh fruits and vegetables, of course!* There's simply no better diet for optimal digestion than one that's filled with raw foods.

Speaking of digestion...

Raw Reason #5: Raw is Easy-to-Digest

Fresh fruits and vegetables are by far the easiest foods to digest.** The main reason for this, as I've already mentioned, is because these foods are full of water and fiber.

In addition, fruits and vegetables are low in fat. Unlike carbohydrates which digest very quickly, fat takes quite a bit more time. Even raw fats like avocados, nuts, and seeds require more time to digest than fruits and vegetables.***

So what does all this mean for you? It means that by going raw, you can finally say goodbye to constipation, diarrhea, bloating, and virtually all other digestive disorders for good!****

Raw Reason #6: Raw is Energizing

---

* Cereal grains like rice and wheat are also full of fiber, but fresh fruit and vegetables are a better source. Check out the next chapter for all the reasons why grains and legumes are subpar foods.

** Cruciferous veggies like broccoli and kale are a bit tougher to digest than tender greens like romaine due to their high cellulose content. If you have trouble digesting these foods raw, try processing them in a blender, food processor, or even with a cheese grater (grated cauliflower makes for delicious raw "rice!"). If that doesn't help, you can steam them slightly first or just avoid them entirely.

*** This is yet another reason why it's best to limit fat intake.

**** To be clear, eating raw doesn't automatically mean you'll have superb digestion. Eating lots of fatty foods, lots of dried foods, and making tons of complicated, dehydrated dishes is a recipe for digestive upset.

Try to think back to a time when you had a really heavy meal. You know, like a steak and potatoes kind of meal.

How did you feel afterwards? I'm willing to bet that the words, sleepy, groggy, and tired come to mind.

Why do we feel so fatigued after a Thanksgiving feast or Fourth of July barbeque? Because digesting food requires energy. The heavier the meal, the more energy it's going to require to fully digest.*

But what if you were to eat a really light meal, like a green smoothie or simple salad? How do you think you would feel then?

It'd probably be a completely different after-meal experience, right? You probably wouldn't have any symptoms of sleepiness—or postprandial somnolence, as it's formally called—at all.

And in fact, that's exactly what raw foodists experience. I honestly cannot remember the last time I felt a drop in energy after a meal! After a healthy raw meal, even a large one that contains 600 calories or more, expect to feel full yet fatigue-free.

In addition to being incredibly easy to digest, a fruit and vegetable-based raw food diet is full of glucose. As I mentioned in chapter two, glucose is the primary fuel source for your cells, *including* your brain cells.

In fact, researchers found that a simple glucose solution (lemonade mixed with sugar) was enough to improve decision-making and self-control![55]

A healthy raw food diet will lessen your digestive load while at the same time provide all of the simple carbohydrates you need to stay alert, energetic, and focused.

---

* Even a relatively "light" meal can evoke this response. I know that when I ate a cooked vegan diet, I often felt sleepy after oatmeal for breakfast, a sandwich for lunch, or another grain- or legume-heavy dish.

Raw Reason #7: Raw is Anti-Obesity

If we were to compare one portion of chicken breast (three ounces) with the same amount of bananas, which do you think would have less calories?

The bananas, of course! Three ounces of chicken breast sans skin is approximately 140 calories while three ounces of bananas is about half of that amount at 76 calories.

But what if we were to compare fresh produce like bananas and romaine with other vegan foods like rice and beans?

Let's have a look.

Table 3.3 Calories in Fruits, Greens, Grains, and Legumes

Food (3 oz)	Calories
Romaine, raw	14 calories
Broccoli, raw	29 calories
Peaches, raw	33 calories
Bananas, raw	76 calories
Brown Rice, cooked	95 calories
Lentils, boiled	99 calories
Whole wheat spaghetti, cooked	105 calories
Barley, cooked	105 calories
Black Beans, boiled	112 calories
Chickpeas, boiled	139 calories

Source: *http://cronometer.com/*

Fresh fruits and vegetables, particularly greens, are clearly lower in calories than grains and legumes. This is great because it means that on a raw food diet centered on fresh fruits and vegetables, you'll get to eat substantially more food without taking in too many calories. You'll be able to lose weight *without* the hassle and discomfort of calorie restriction.

In fact, some raw foodists like myself find that they're able to eat *more* calories (sometimes significantly more) on a raw food diet while weighing *less* than they ever did eating predominantly cooked foods!

Sounds crazy, but there are a few likely reasons for this.

#1: Fiber

Unlike animal products, raw fruits and vegetables are full of fiber. Fiber is great for digestion, but little to none of it (depending upon the type of fiber) is actually absorbed by the body.

In other words, fiber has virtually no calories!

#2: Thermogenesis

The second concept that may explain why some people can consume more calories on a raw food diet is something called thermogenesis. As Dr. Colin T. Campbell explains in *The China Study*:

> **Consuming diets *high* in protein and fat transfers calories away from their conversion into body heat to their storage form—as body fat (unless severe calorie restriction is causing weight loss). In contrast, diets *low* in protein and fat cause calories to be 'lost' as body heat.[56]**

In other words, you burn slightly more calories on a low protein, high carbohydrate diet and a healthy raw vegan diet is low in protein and high in carbs.

#3: Body Temperature

The third and final possible reason why weight gain is more difficult on raw foods has to do with body temperature. Many people experience a slightly lower body temperature after switching to a raw food diet, probably due to less body fat and the fact that no warm or hot foods are consumed.

What does a lower body temperature have to do with weight loss? When you're cold, your body has to work to warm you up. This extra work burns extra calories.[*58] We also tend to move around more when we're cold in an attempt to warm up. More movement means more calories burned.

Regardless of whether or not you're able to eat more calories than when you ate a cooked food diet, eating a raw food diet focused on low-calorie, nutritious fruits and vegetables makes reaching and maintaining an ideal weight virtually effortless.[**]

Raw Reason #8: Raw is Anti-Disease

Any advice not recognizing that raw vegetables and fresh fruits are the two most powerful anti-cancer categories of foods is off the mark. ~ Dr. Joel Fuhrman, Eat To Live[59]

Dr. Fuhrman is absolutely right. Consumption of fresh fruit and vegetables has been associated with a decreased risk for numerous cancers, including:

- Bladder cancer[60-61]
- Breast cancer[60-61]
- Cervical cancer[60-61]
- Colorectal cancer[60-61]
- Esophageal cancer[60-61]
- Kidney cancer[62]
- Lung cancer[61]
- Oral cancer[60-61]
- Ovarian cancer[60-61]
- Pancreatic cancer[60-61]
- Prostate cancer[61]
- Stomach cancer[60-61]

And it's not just cancer that fresh produce protects against. Eating fruits and vegetables has been linked to a decreased risk for several noncancerous diseases and disorders, including:

---

* In *The 4-Hour Body*, author Tim Ferris recommends ice baths as a weight loss strategy![57]

** The best way to determine your ideal weight is to focus on body fat percentage and waist-to-height ratio, not the number on the scale. For body fat percentage, women should aim for high teens to low twenties and men should aim for low to high teens. Slightly lower is likely okay, but is often difficult to maintain without constant calorie restriction. For waist-to-height ratio, both men and women should aim for a waist circumference that's less than half of their height.

- Cardiovascular disease[63]
- Cataracts[63]
- Chronic obstructive pulmonary disease (COPD)[63]
- Diabetes mellitus (type II)[63]
- Macular degeneration[63]
- Obesity[64-66]
- Osteoporosis[64]

Combine this with all the health benefits that come with avoiding animal products, processed carbs, and large amounts of fat and you've got one incredibly healthy, disease-resistant diet!*

Raw Reason #9: Raw is Alkaline-Forming

Unlike animal products and grains, fresh fruits and vegetables are alkaline-forming foods.** Eating lots of these potassium-rich foods has been linked to the preservation of muscle mass as well as the prevention of bone loss and hip fractures.[68, 69-70]

Vitamin K may also be protective against poor bone health. Vitamin K is necessary for osteocalin, a protein that helps bones resist fracture, to get absorbed into your bones.[71] Fruits and vegetables, particularly leafy greens, are the best sources of vitamin K.

Raw Reason #10: Raw is Good for the Planet

There's no doubt that a raw vegan diet is incredibly eco-friendly.

For one, it's completely devoid of animals products. As I talked about in chapter one, livestock production is incredibly damaging to the environment and is one of the leading causes of air and water pollution, deforestation, soil erosion, and loss of biodiversity.[72]

A diet focused on fresh fruits and veggies also requires less packaging than processed food items. No bottles, cans, or jars and very little plastic or cardboard is used.

---

* In fact, fruits and vegetables alone may not do much to lower cancer risk as a whole.[67] Eating healthfully is just as much about what you don't eat (meat, dairy, and processed carbs) as it is about what you do eat (fruits and vegetables).

** While citrus fruits like oranges and lemons are acidic, they are not metabolized to acidic compounds. Therefore, they are alkalizing foods.

Plus, the fruits and veggies themselves are actually *good* for the environment. Fruit trees are especially beneficial since they "heal the environment by cleaning the air, improving soil quality, preventing erosion, creating animal habitat" and "sustaining valuable water sources." (*http://www.ftpf.org/*) And left over peels and such can easily be composted for an eco-friendly (and economical) home garden.

Fruits and Vegetables for the Win!

There's no doubt that a raw food diet based on fresh fruits and vegetables is an amazing way to eat. To recap, a healthy raw food diet.

- is low in calories, fat, and toxins;
- is full of vitamins, minerals, water, and fiber;
- brings you superior digestion and abundant energy;
- significantly reduces your risk for obesity, cancer, and numerous other diseases;
- and is good for you and the planet!

And there are so many other benefits to eating raw that I haven't even mentioned! A raw food diet done right often means

- no more acne, psoriasis, keratosis pilaris, or other skin conditions;
- no more migraines or headaches;
- better sleep;
- healthier, hair;
- much less body odor;
- and much more mental clarity!

Now only one question remains: what exactly is a raw food diet done right? Don't worry, chapter five is all about showing you the right way to go raw. First, I need to explain why all raw foods are NOT equal.

CHAPTER 4
All Raw Foods Are Not Equal

As you probably noticed while reading the last chapter, I often equate raw foods with fresh fruits and vegetables. That's because on a healthy, nutritionally complete raw food diet, that's what will make up the vast majority of your diet: fresh fruits and vegetables.

Besides, just saying "eat raw food" is misleading. By that logic, anything raw is fair game. The grass in your backyard is raw. Should you eat it? Poison ivy is raw as well. Should you snack on that, too?

Of course not!

That said, there are raw foods that many raw foodists eat that may not be healthy for us. Buckwheat greens, which can cause sensitivity to sunlight as well as other skin issues, is one example.[1] Irish moss, a red seaweed that causes inflammation due to the presence of carrageenan, is another one.[2]

The real issue is whether or not the food in question is suited for human consumption. In other words, we want to know whether or not it is nutrient-rich, low in toxins, and palatable.

Luckily, the philosophy of Natural Hygiene provides us with an easy way to figure all of this out. Taste the food in its whole, raw state without any condiments. What does it taste like? Is it palatable? Is it satisfying? Could you eat an entire bowl of it?

By applying this simple test, you'll find that many so-called healthy foods are not an appropriate foodstuff for humans. Grains, legumes, and tubers like potatoes and yams are perfect examples, as they are inedible when raw. These foods must be prepared in some way—either by soaking, sprouting, fermenting, or cooking—to make them palatable and digestible.

In addition, these foods are not very appealing in their whole state. Even when sprouted or cooked, foods like rice and pinto beans still require flavor enhancers like salt, spices, and sauces to make them tasty.

Palatability aside, there are several reasons why grains, legumes, and tubers are not ideal foods.

Grains

Anti-Nutrients

While all plant foods contain some anti-nutrients like phytates (phytic acid) and lectins, grains contain higher amounts than fruits and vegetables.* This is of concern because anti-nutrients inhibit your body's absorption of certain minerals like calcium and iron.

Below I'll discuss the four main anti-nutrients—phytic acid, lectins, tannins, and enzyme inhibitors—present in grains and their effects on human health.

Phytic Acid

It's well-known that phytic acid significantly inhibits calcium, iron, magnesium, manganese and zinc absorption.[5-9] One study found that when male subjects were fed wheat rolls containing 2, 25, and 250 mg of phytic acid, iron absorption was decreased by 18, 64, and 82 percent!**[6]

It's no wonder that the World Health Organization (WHO) considers high phytate intake one of the main causes of iron deficiency anaemia.***[10]

---

* Nuts and seeds are also high in phytates and lectins and have been shown to inhibit iron absorption.[3,4] This is yet another reason to limit your consumption of nuts and seeds.

** It's important to note that adding ascorbic acid (vitamin C) to the subjects' meals "significantly counteracted the inhibition" of iron.[6] For more information on vitamin C and iron absorption, please see chapter six.

*** I struggled with anaemia for many years and found that my symptoms were at their worst when I was on a grain and legume-heavy vegetarian diet.

Phytic acid has also been shown to inhibit, protein, lipid, and starch absorption.[11-13]

Lectin

Lectin is a carbohydrate-binding protein that binds to the lining of the intestines and can cause intestinal damage when consumed in high amounts.* This results in compromised absorption of various nutrients and can cause inflammation and gut permeability in those sensitive to lectin.[14-17]

This permeability allows the lectins to enter your bloodstream and attach themselves to your vital tissues. Your body then attacks the lectins and the tissues they are attached to, which may contribute to autoimmune diseases like rheumatoid arthritis.[18]

Lectins may also contribute to weight gain by disrupting leptin, a hormone that regulates hunger, and anxiety and depression as well.[19, 20]

Tannins

Barley and sorghum are high in tannins, which are bitter-tasting polyphenolic compounds found in many plants.** Tannins bind to protein and certain minerals thereby reducing digestibility of these nutrients.[21-22]

Enzyme Inhibitors

Grains like rice contain enzyme inhibitors that are "believed to cause growth inhibition by interfering with digestion, causing pancreatic hypertrophy [enlargement] and metabolic disturbance of sulfur amino acid utilization."[23]

---

* Nightshade plants, which include tomatoes, potatoes, and eggplant, are also high in lectins. While potatoes and eggplant are typically avoided on a raw food diet, tomatoes are delicious when eaten raw. However, if you are particularly sensitive to lectins (i.e. you suffer from IBS, celiac disease, joint inflammation, etc.), you may find it useful to limit or even eliminate tomatoes from your diet.

** It's the high tannin content in unripe Hachiya persimmons that gives the fruit it's bitter taste and astringency. You'll know when the Hachiya is ripe because it becomes very soft and super sweet!

Grains & Gluten

Wheat, barley, and rye all contain gluten, a protein responsible for the chewy texture of dough.* Unfortunately, that's not all for which gluten is responsible.

Gastrointestinal Disorders

When people with celiac disease consume wheat, barley, or rye, the gluten in these grains damages the lining of their small intestines and inhibits nutrient absorption. This can then cause abdominal pain, diarrhea, nausea, weight loss, depression, fatigue, hair loss, and seizures.[24]

But even people without celiac disease can suffer from gluten intolerance (aka gluten sensitivity).[25-28] Dr. Daniel Leffler, an assistant professor of medicine at Harvard Medical School, estimates that half of Americans who suffer from irritable bowel syndrome (IBS) are sensitive to gluten.[29] Dr. Alessio Fasano, medical director of the University of Maryland for Celiac Research, estimates that 18 million Americans suffer from at least some form of gluten sensitivity.[30]

These estimates are at least partially verified by the growing number of people who have given up gluten and experienced marked improvements in digestion as a result.[31-36]

Autism

The link between autism and GI disorders is well-known. One study found that 45% of children with autism spectrum disorders (ASDs) showed gastrointestinal symptoms such as abdominal pain, constipation, and diarrhea.[37]

Another study analyzing over 41,000 children from 3 to 17 years old found that the children with autism were *seven times* more likely to suffer from frequent diarrhea and colitis than the children without any developmental disability![38-39]

---

* While oats themselves are gluten-free, they're often contaminated with gluten due to being grown or processed with wheat and barley.

So it makes sense that gluten, which is clearly connected to GI disorders, is also linked to autism. In fact, researchers and parents have found that switching children with autism to a gluten/casein-free diet leads to improvements in social behavior.[40-42]

Autoimmune Disease

In addition to celiac disease, gluten has been linked to numerous autoimmune disorders, including rheumatoid arthritis, Hashimoto's thyroiditis, type 1 diabetes, and systemic lupus erythematosus (SLE).*[43-44, 45, 46-47, 48]

Depression

Gluten has also been linked to depression, with one study finding that about one-third of subjects with celiac disease also suffered from depression.[49, 50]

Grains & Fiber

Grains and fiber? But fiber is good for you, right?

There are two types of fiber: insoluble fiber and soluble fiber. Fruits, vegetables, grains, and legumes all contain both insoluble and soluble fiber, but in varying amounts. Fruits tend to be higher in soluble fiber while grains and legumes are higher in insoluble fiber. Vegetables are also higher in insoluble fiber, but they generally contain more soluble fiber than grains and legumes do.

What's the big deal? The big deal is that while soluble fiber (will dissolve in water) is very soft and easy on your digestive tract, insoluble fiber (won't dissolve in water) can be rather rough.

How rough? I'll let cell biologist Dr. Paul L. McNeil describe it for you:

---

* My mom used to suffer from arthritic symptoms, especially during the winter months when her joints would become very stiff and painful. Giving up gluten has completely eliminated these symptoms. Eating gluten for just a couple days in a row is enough to bring some pain back into her hands.

When you eat high fiber foods [such as grains and fibers that can't be completely digested], they bang up against the cells lining the gastrointestinal tract, rupturing their outer covering...this banging and tearing increases the level of lubricating mucus.[51]

According to Dr. McNeil, the fact that insoluble fiber injures your cells and increases mucus production is a good thing because it "promotes health of the GI tract as a whole."[51] I'm not so sure.

In fact, I suspect that it's this "banging and tearing" that's partly to blame for Irritable Bowel Syndrome (IBS), Crohn's disease, and other debilitating digestive disorders afflicting so many grain-eaters today.[*]

In addition, fruits and vegetables have been implicated again and again in protection against colorectal cancer, one of the most common types of cancer in the United States.[53-56] While cereal fiber has also shown to be protective against colorectal cancer, the results have been mixed and more and more studies are showing vegetable fiber to be more protective.[53, 55, 57]

As Dr. John D. Potter writes in "Dietary Fiber, Vegetables, and Cancer":

...if there is a place for a specific message at this time in the unfolding relationship between diet and colorectal cancer it is not "eat more fiber" but "eat more vegetables.[58]

Finally, the high amounts of insoluble fiber present in grains may be partly "responsible for poor digestibility of protein" in these foods.[12]

Fiber is important, but you don't need grains to get it and you certainly don't need the "banging and tearing" or "mucus production" that results from eating these foods. A raw food diet sufficient in fruits and vegetables will supply all the soluble and insoluble fiber you need for optimal digestion.

---

[*]   My belief is supported by many former IBS sufferers who have been able to cure themselves by giving up grains.[52]

Grains & Opioids

Dairy products aren't the only foods that contain addictive opioids. Cereal grains like wheat and barley do, too![59-61]

Melissa Diane Smith, author of *Going Against the Grain: How Reducing and Avoiding Grains Can Revitalize Your Health* writes:

> Opioid substances have a very similar sequence of amino acids to those in our natural endorphins and apparently can bind to endorphin receptors in the brain. They also have a very similar sequence of amino acids to those in addictive, narcotic-like drugs—exorphins literally mean morphine-like molecules that come from the outside environment. In simple terms, exorphins produce narcotic-like and mood-altering effects and can be addictive.[62]

This may explain why so many people find it so difficult to give up grain-heavy foods like pasta and bread.

Grains & Acidosis

Like animal products, grains are acid-forming and play a role in metabolic acidosis.[63-64]

Grains vs. Fruits and Veggies

Grains are simply a subpar food when compared to fruits and vegetables. They contain less nutrients per calories and more toxins like phytic acid, lectins, and opioids. They're also acid-forming, high in rough insoluble fiber, and have been linked to numerous digestive disorders.

They may be better than meat and milk, but even whole grains can't compete with fresh fruits and veggies.

What About Sprouted Grains?

While sprouting has little effect on gluten-containing grains, it does improve starch and protein digestibility, destroy enzyme inhibitors, decreases phytic acid, and increase the bio-availability of certain nutrients.[65, 66, 67-68]

So if you'd like to include raw grains in your diet, it's definitely best to sprout them first. Avoiding grains with gluten and focusing on brown rice, gluten-free oats, and pseudo-grains like wild rice, quinoa, and amaranth is also recommended.

Legumes

Legumes & Anti-Nutrients

Like grains, legumes contain more anti-nutrients than fruits and vegetables. They're high in phytates and enzyme inhibitors that can interfere with your body's own digestive enzymes.[3 & 69, 70-71]

Legumes also contain high amounts of lectins like hemagglutinins.[72] Red kidney beans are particularly high in hemagglutinins and, unless cooked properly, can result in "extreme" nausea, vomiting, and diarrhea.[73]

Legumes & Oligosaccharides

Beans, beans, the musical fruit... Oh, you know the story. But did you ever wonder why beans and other legumes make us so...musical?

Blame it on the oligosaccharides.

Oligosaccharide is a complex sugar found in legumes. Because humans do not posses the enzymes necessary to break down this sugar, the large molecules are able to pass through our digestive systems mostly intact. Once the sugars reach our large intestines, they ferment in the presence of bacteria and give us gas.[74-75]

Legumes vs. Fruits and Veggies

Although gluten-free, opioid-free, and more nutrient-dense than grains, legumes are still a subpar food. They're acid-forming, high in insoluble fiber, contain indigestible sugars, and have higher amounts of anti-nutrients than fresh fruits and vegetables.

What About Sprouted Legumes?

Sprouting legumes improves starch and protein digestibility, destroys enzyme inhibitors (becoming raw), decreases lectins and phytic acid, and increases the bio-availability of certain nutrients. It also reduces the amount of oligosaccharide and hemagglutinin.[1 & 76]

Like raw grains, it's best to sprout raw legumes if you wish to include them in your diet. However, kidney beans should never be consumed raw due to the high amount of hemagglutinin they contain.

Tubers

Other than cassava, which contains cyanogenic glucosides, most tubers contain low amounts of toxins.[*][77] Potato, sweet potato, and yam are all low in phytic acid and lower in lectins and enzyme inhibitors than grains and legumes.[3] Plus, the majority of these anti-nutrients are in the skin, which can easily be peeled away and discarded.[77]

Potatoes do contain glycoalkaloids that are not destroyed during cooking, but the amount is low in commercial varieties.[77] Potatoes also contain hemagglutinins which are destroyed when cooked.[77]

---

[*]   Cyanogenic glucoside is a toxin that can transform into the poison hydrogen cyanide when consumed.

Tubers vs. Fruits and Veggies

Although not as offensive as grains and legumes, tubers can't compete with fruits and vegetables. They're starchy and difficult to digest unless cooked, contain toxins like glycoalkaloids and hemagglutinins, and are not as nutrient-dense as fresh fruits and green vegetables.

What About Sprouted Tubers?

There really isn't any reason to eat sprouted potatoes, sweet potatoes, or yams. In fact, potatoes that have sprouted should never be consumed because they contain higher amounts of glycoalkaloids.[78]

If you want to consume tubers, cooking them first is really the best choice.*

What About Raw Animal Products?

You already learned from chapter one that there are many downsides to eating meat, milk, and other animal products. To recap, these food items are:

- **high in cholesterol;**
- **high in saturated fat;**
- **high in protein;****
- **low in fiber;**
- **associated with a whole host of human diseases including heart disease, diabetes, and various cancers;**
- **full of harmful contaminants such as dioxins, hormones, pesticides, and opioids**
- **a serious burden on the environment; and**
- **the result of torture and death for an unfathomable number of**

---

*   That said, raw sweet potato does make for a really delicious, crunchy, oil-free chip. Just thinly slice the potato, sprinkle on some paprika, dehydrate for a few hours, and devour with your favorite raw dip!

**   Remember, excess protein is hard on your kidneys and has been linked to various life-threatening illnesses.

cows, pigs, chickens, sheep, fish, and other domesticated animals.

Now you may be wondering: aren't animal products like meat and milk typically eaten when cooked, as in roasted chicken, scrambled eggs, or pasteurized milk? Could eating these foods raw perhaps make a difference?

Raw Meat is Still Meat

Throwing a steak on the grill or a chicken in the oven doesn't change the fact that these foods are still animal products. Raw or not, steak, chicken, and other meats are chock full of cholesterol, completely free of fiber, and brimming with bacteria.

Is Raw Worth the Risk?

By consuming raw animal products, you would avoid carcinogens such as HCAs that are created when these foods are heated. On the other hand, you would be susceptible to higher levels of bacteria such as *E. coli* and *Salmonella* that would not be destroyed during the cooking process.

This is perfectly fine for carnivores like tigers, wolves, and other species that have very strong gastric acid that can kill this bacteria, but it is not fine for us. Our stomach acid is much milder and our digestive tracts much longer, allowing the bacteria to live on and make us sick, sometimes fatally so.[79-80]

Humans Are Not Carnivores

A brief look at human anatomy and physiology will tell you that our species is most certainly not suited for consuming meat and milk. As I already mentioned, humans have shorter digestive tracts and milder gastric acid than those of carnivores.

In addition, we have:

- flat teeth that are good for grinding;[81]
- lateral jaw movement that's also good for grinding; [81]
- digestive enzymes in our saliva; [81]
- a liver that cannot detoxify vitamin A; [81] and
- flat nails that are good for grasping. [81]

Carnivores are quite different. They have sharp teeth and claws that are great for ripping and tearing, very little side-to-side jaw mobility, no digestive enzymes in their saliva, and livers that can detoxify vitamin A.[*] [81]

Anthropologists Agree: Our Ancestors Were Mostly Vegetarian

Paleo dieters, those who follow a meat-heavy diet supposedly modeled after the diets of our paleolithic ancestors, will argue that we relied on meat for the majority of human existence and, therefore, meat is our ideal fuel source.[**]

The truth is likely quite different. In fact, most experts agree that our ancestors were mostly vegetarian, subsisting on fruit, nuts, leaves, and small amounts of insects and animal flesh.[***][83, 84]

Cow Milk is for Calves

Milk is nourishment for baby mammals. Once the animal reaches a certain age, it no longer requires mother's milk . As a result, its body stops producing lactase, the enzyme that breaks down the milk sugar lactose.

---

[*] The ability to detoxify vitamin A is very important since vitamin A is a fat-soluble vitamin (your body can store it) and is found in high amounts in animal products. For more on the dangers of consuming vitamin A from animal products, pleas see chapter six.

[**] While our ancestors certainly consumed meat, it's important to note that the wild game our ancestors consumed was very different from our modern-day domestic meats. It was naturally lower in saturated fat and omega-6s, higher in omega-3s, and may have resulted in less inflammation as well.[82]

[***] In college, many of my anthropology professors made it clear that our hunter-gatherer ancestors were gatherers first and hunters second, with about 70% of the diet made up of foraged foods. One of my professors even referred to them as gatherer-hunters!

Humans are different, you say? Yes and no.

While it's true that many adults today are big milk drinkers, it wasn't always this way. Prior to animal domestication, humans were weaned from their mother's milk in infancy just like all other mammals.[85]

Thanks to thousands of years of milk-chugging by our central and northern European ancestors, most Westerners today continue to produce lactase throughout their entire lives.*[86]

So doesn't this suggest that drinking milk as an adult is actually a healthy practice for those of us who aren't lactose intolerant?

Not really. As I explained in chapter one, milk and other dairy products are high in calories, saturated fat, and cholesterol; completely devoid of fiber; and have been linked to numerous diseases and disorders.

Conclusion

Not all raw foods are equal. Some, like grains and legumes, contain high amounts of anti-nutrients. Others, like meat and dairy, are full of fat and cholesterol.

Now this doesn't mean that a raw food diet that contains some of these products is automatically unhealthy. What you eat in small amounts and infrequently likely won't have much of an impact as long as the majority of your diet is made up of two very important ingredients: fresh fruits and vegetables.

---

* Lactose intolerance remains very common amongst people whose ancestors did not consume milk. For instance, about 90% of Asian-American adults are lactose intolerant.[87]

CHAPTER 5
The Best Raw Food Diet for Health and Vitality

As I said in the introduction to this book, the raw food movement needs a facelift. For far too long, the message has been "Give up cooked foods, eat raw, and voila!"

This chapter is all about eating raw the right way so you can lose weight, feel great, and experience the best health of your life.

But first...

The Worst Raw Food Diet

We already know from chapter two that filling up on fat is a bad idea. Excess fat in the diet is linked to inflammation, insulin resistance, immune suppression, and weight gain.

And yet, this is what many raw foodists are doing every single day! They're filling up on fatty foods like avocados, nuts, seeds, and oils at the expense of the only other fuel source on a raw food diet: fresh fruit.

Why? Because raw foodists are afraid of fruit.

Why? Because certain raw food educators are telling them that fruit isn't such a great food.

Why? Because "too much" fruit will spike your blood sugar, give you cancer, promote candidiasis, damage your liver, ruin your teeth, and make you fat.

Wait, what?!

Fruit is Not the Enemy

My main goal for this chapter is to prove to you why fruit is such a healthy food and why including it in your diet is absolutely vital to your success with raw foods. In order to do that, I have to start by dispelling all of the common fruit fallacies I mentioned above.

Fruit Fallacy #1: Fruit is High-Glycemic

The glycemic index (GI) measures how quickly particular foods are digested and how quickly the sugars in those foods enter into the bloodstream. The sugars in a food with a high GI (above 70) quickly enter the bloodstream causing a more rapid rise in blood glucose levels.

Most fruits actually have a low to medium GI (1-55 is low, 56-69 is medium). Watermelon and pineapple are two exceptions.[*][1]

In any event, glycemic index isn't the end-all-be-all. In fact, eating foods based solely on the glycemic index is an easy way to ensure unhealthy eating. M&M's with peanuts, Betty Crocker chocolate cake (including the oh-so healthy chocolate frosting), Pizza Hut "super supreme" pizza, and Twix Cookie Bars all have a low GI.[1]

Fruit Fallacy #2: Fruit Spikes Your Blood Sugar

It's true that when you eat fruit, the level of sugar in your blood rises and then comes back down sometime later. In fact, this is what happens every time you eat, no matter what you eat!

It could be hot dogs or it could be a salad with oil and vinegar. Eating food will raise your blood sugar and your body will have to work to lower it again.

---

[*] The glycemic index only measures the rate at which the sugar in a food enters the bloodstream, not the amount of sugar in a particular amount of food. This is where the glycemic load (GL) comes in. Virtually all fresh fruit, including high GI species like pineapple and watermelon, have a low GL (10 or below).[1]

The important thing is how quickly your blood sugar returns to normal. With most difficult-to-digest foods eaten on a standard American diet of fatty meats and refined grains, this process is rather slow.

On the other hand, fruit digests quickly and easily. Within just minutes after eating a meal of fruit, your body will already have started the process of transporting the sugar out of your blood and into your cells.

So yes, eating fruit raises your blood sugar. Is this a bad thing? Not at all. In fact, it's simply a necessary part of eating! As long as blood sugar does not remain elevated and does not go above the accepted range (70-130 mg/dL fasting, less than 180 mg/dL two hours after a meal), you have nothing to worry about.[2]

If you still don't believe that eating a diet high in fruit won't spike your blood sugar, you can easily test it for yourself with a glucose meter and testing strips bought at your local convenience or grocery store.[*]

Diabetes and Fruit

What if you suffer from type II diabetes? How can you possibly eat fruit without your blood sugar skyrocketing out of control?

Unfortunately, most people are taught once a diabetic, always a diabetic. The truth is that type II diabetes CAN be reversed, as Dr. Neal Barnard proves in his life-saving book *Dr. Neal Barnard's Program for Reversing Diabetes*.

How does he do it? He does it with a low fat, low glycemic, high carbohydrate vegan diet.

This really is no surprise, given what we learned about fat and insulin resistance in chapter two. Remember, it's excess fat in the diet accompanied with sugar that causes blood sugar spikes, not the sugar alone.

---

[*] I've taken my own blood glucose on numerous occasions eating a low fat, high fruit diet and have never had an abnormal reading. Both my fasting blood sugar (no food for at least 8 hours) and my postprandial blood sugar (two hours after a meal) have always been well within the normal ranges. Here's a video of my taking my blood sugar after a giant fruit-packed green smoothie: **http://www.fitonraw.com/2011/11/what-really-happens-after-a-big-fruit-meal/**

Cut back on the fat and you should have no problem digesting and absorbing as much fruit as you care to consume.[*]

Fruit Fallacy #3: Fruit Causes Cancer

This myth stems from the fact that sugar feeds cancer cells and fruit, of course, is full of sugar. The fact is, sugar feeds *all* cells and *any* food you eat will eventually be converted to glucose. So if you have cancer and you eat food, you will feed the cancerous cells in your body.[**]

This is likely why fasting is proving to be such an effective cancer treatment.[6-9] When you fast, you don't take in any food so there is nothing to fuel the cancer cells.

But let's get back to the question at hand. Does fruit actually *cause* cancer?

There is absolutely no evidence that this is so. In fact, as I showed in chapter three, study after study after study has shown that the people who include *more* fruit in their diet are at a *lower* risk for various cancers, along with other life-threatening diseases like diabetes and heart disease.

In fact, the American Cancer Association recommends that fruit be included in *every meal* as part of its dietary guidelines for cancer prevention![10]

Fruit Fallacy #4: Fruit Causes Liver Damage

[*]   Avoiding high-glycemic fruits (watermelon and pineapple) and including greens along with your fruit may help slow down sugar uptake. Also, you may want to consider taking a chromium supplement since chromium is necessary for blood sugar metabolism. According to long-term raw foodist Don Bennett, some of the people with diabetes who he has coached were unable to completely eliminate their need insulin until they began supplementing with chromium.[3] For more information on chromium and other supplements, stay tuned for chapter seven.

[**]   That's not to say that a fruit- and vegetable-rich diet wouldn't be good for those struggling with cancer. For one thing, these foods are full of water and water is necessary for proper blood oxygenation. Hypoxia, or low oxygen levels, may contribute to tumor growth.[4-5] Plus, fruits and vegetables contain apigenin that has "growth inhibitory properties in several cancer lines, including breast, colon, skin, thyroid, and leukemia cells" and has been shown to "inhibit pancreatic cancer cell proliferation."[6]

This fallacy stems from the fact that fruit contains fructose. Fructose is a simple sugar processed primarily by the liver, one of the byproducts of which is a fat called triglyceride. An excess of triglycerides in the body has been linked to hepatic steatosis (nonalcoholic fatty liver disease), as well as heart disease and stroke.[11-13, 14, 15-16]

So why am I not concerned about all of the fructose in fruit? Because all of the studies linking fructose to disease refer only to *refined* fructose, typically in the form of High Fructose Corn Syrup (HFCS) or fruit juices.[17-23] To my knowledge, there isn't a single study that links fresh fruit to liver damage of any kind.

And as I already mentioned, fruit is recommended for cancer prevention. Some studies have even shown that the more fruits and vegetables you consume, the lower your risk for liver cancer.[24-25]

Even Mr. Anti-Fructose himself Dr. Robert Lustig admits that it is refined fructose that's dangerous, not fructose from fresh fruit that still has its fiber intact.[*26]

Fruit Fallacy #5: Fruit Causes *Candida* Overgrowth

Candida is nothing more than a group of yeast that live on your skin and in your mouth. It's completely normal and is kept in check by the presence of other bacteria as well as your own white blood cells.

Candida overgrowth, or candidiasis, is a condition in which the *Candida* has been allowed to proliferate. This usually occurs in warm and moist areas like the mouth, underarms, under the breasts, under the nails, or in and around the genitalia.[27]

So what causes candidiasis?

Unsurprisingly, candidiasis typically occurs in people taking antibiotics

---

* I've been consuming the vast majority of my calories from fruit and taking in tons of fructose since 2007, yet my liver is in great condition. According to some blood work I had done in June 2012, my triglycerides were well below threshold (80 mg/dl) and my AST, ALT, APT, and bilirubin (tests used to check liver function) were all within the normal ranges. I even made a video showing all of my blood work from 2012, which you can see here: *http://www.fitonraw.com/2012/07/my-low-fat-raw-vegan-blood-test-results/*

or steroids, which destroy the bacteria that help stop *Candida* from proliferating.* It's also commonly seen in people who are overweight or suffering from diabetes or immunodeficiency disorders like leukemia and AIDS.[27 & 29]

And how do you know if you have candidiasis?

According to the alternative medical community, candidiasis has many symptoms including headaches, migraines, depression, insomnia, fatigue, dizziness, irritability, numbness, anxiety, hypoglycemia, bloating, constipation, asthma, joint pain, premenstrual syndrome (PMS), and infertility.[30-32]

No wonder we're all so afraid of *Candida*!

In truth, candidiasis is a fungal infection and is fairly easily diagnosed. For instance, thrush (oral candidiasis) is characterized by white lesions covering the tongue.[33] Vaginal yeast infections involve itching, burning, and abnormal vaginal discharge.[34]

If you have all the "symptoms" of candidiasis but have no signs of a fungal infection, you probably don't have candidiasis. Feeling anxious, bloated, or fatigued can be caused by any number of things that have nothing to do with *Candida*, including too much stress, a fatty diet, or just lack of sleep!

But If I Eat Fruit, Won't I Get Candidiasis?

The reason fruit gets the blame for causing *Candida* overgrowth is because *Candida* feeds on sugar.** Fruit, of course, is full of sugar.

Sounds scary, but it really isn't.

---

* Women who douche are also more likely to get *Candida* overgrowth in the form of vaginal yeast infections.[28]

** Many low fat, high fruit raw vegans also support the alternative model of candidiasis (i.e. candidiasis and even systemic Candidiasis are common place), but they believe the cause to be a fat-filled diet instead of a sugar-filled one (i.e. fat slows down sugar absorption so the *Candida* in your blood has more fuel to live on and proliferate). I once believed this as well and even wrote an entire article blaming candidiasis on fat. While there may indeed be a connection between Candida overgrowth and fat intake (e.g. type II diabetics often suffer from Candidiasis and type II diabetes is linked to high-fat diets), clinical evidence shows that systemic Candidiasis is not common place at all, but is in fact very rare and very deadly.

Remember that *Candida* exists *outside* of the body on your skin and in your mouth. If *Candida* does enter the bloodstream—through a cut on your finger, for instance—your white blood cells will attack it and stop the yeast from proliferating.

If the *Candida does* proliferate—which it can in those suffering from AIDS, leukemia, or some other immunodeficiency disorder—it can infect the entire body, a condition known as systemic candidiasis (candidemia). Although rare, systemic candidiasis is a very serious and even deadly condition.[27]

In other words, the fact that fruit is full of sugar really doesn't matter. Unless you have systemic candidiasis, there won't be any *Candida* in your bloodstream to feed on the sugar anyway!

So in conclusion, fruit does not cause candidiasis. If you feel fatigued, bloated, anxious, or any of the other candidiasis "symptoms," it most likely isn't because of a *Candida* overgrowth.

On the other hand, if you have thrush, a vaginal yeast infection, or some other skin infection that a medical doctor has diagnosed as candidiasis, this has nothing to do with "too much" fruit in your diet. It's very likely the result of antibiotic or steroid use, diabetes, excess body fat, or just plain bad hygiene.

Fruit Fallacy #6: Fruit Causes Tooth Decay

This fruit myth is pretty easy to understand. Fruit is full of sugar and sugar causes cavities...or does it?

The truth is, sugar isn't really the issue when it comes to tooth decay. As Dr. Robert Nara explains in *Money by the Mouthful*, it's germs that are to blame.[35]

Having healthy teeth is not about avoiding sweets or visiting your dentist every six months. It's about following a regular routine that keeps your teeth clean and the bacteria in your mouth in a disorganized state.

How do you do this? By following a good dental hygiene program. Specifically I mean brushing morning and night, flossing daily, and using some kind of anti-bacterial rinse at night (e.g. ACT Fluoride Rinse, clove oil, etc.).*

I also highly recommend disclosing tablets, which contain a dye that stains any plaque on your teeth bright red. It's a great way to test your brushing and flossing skills.

Fruit Fallacy #7: Fruit Makes You Fat

This one is true simply because *any* food has the potential to pack on the pounds if you eat enough of it.** If you consume more calories than you need, no matter if it's cantaloupe or cookies, you will gain body fat.

For most people, consuming too many calories from fruit will be pretty difficult simply because fruit is so full of water and fiber. You'll feel fuller on less calories than you would eating more concentrated and fiber-free foods like meat and processed carbohydrates.

This is why most people find it so easy to reach a healthy weight following a fruit-centered raw food diet. For the few people who do struggle with weight gain on a high- fruit diet, the answer is simple: you're eating too much fruit.

Why do you feel the need to overeat? The most likely reason is that you aren't fulfilling all of your nutritional needs, which can happen if you focus too much on fruit at the expense of greens and other vegetables.**

---

* After brushing with only water for a few years, my teeth became pretty yellow. I also found that it took quite a bit of time to remove all of the plaque from my teeth. Now I use a toothpowder when I brush, which has made my teeth much whiter and easier to clean. My favorite brand is Eco-Dent.

** I personally found this to be the case for me. When my vegetable intake was low, I needed over 2500 calories from fruit to feel satiated. This added excess weight to my body and left me feeling bloated and uncomfortable. As soon as I started eating more vegetables, I was able to lower my caloric intake significantly and lose the excess body fat.

Fruit is Your Friend

If you're going to succeed with a raw food lifestyle, you have to eat lots of fruit.* The only way you can consume enough calories to maintain a healthy weight and meet your nutrient needs *without* overdoing it on fat is by focusing on fruit.

Why? Because there are only two sources of calories on a raw food diet: fruit or fatty foods like avocados, nuts, seeds, mature coconut meat, and oils.

What about vegetables like broccoli and spinach? Foods like these are simply too low in calories to provide the fuel your body needs. For instance, a full pound of romaine lettuce contains *less than* 100 calories!

On the other hand, a varied diet of fresh fruit contains plenty of calories for the average adult, while still being high in water and fiber, full of necessary vitamins and minerals, low in toxins, easy to digest, and extremely satiating.

Fun Fruit Facts

Did you know that bananas are just as good as sports drinks for athletic performance? And according to head researcher Dr. David C. Neiman, bananas had numerous advantages, including their antioxidant, fiber, potassium, and vitamin B6 content.[36]

Did you know that fruit is full of folate, an important B vitamin that may help treat depression?[37]

Did you know that fruit can significantly reduce your risk for esophageal cancer, larynx cancer, and oral cancer?[38]

Did you know that watermelon is rich in citrulline, an amino acid that

---

* Success is not just defined by how long you stay raw. It's also defined by the state of your health. While some raw foodists are able to stay raw for years eating lots of avocados, nuts, seeds, and oils, this doesn't mean they are healthy.

has proven to be an effective treatment for mild to moderate erectile dysfunction?[39]

Did you know that fruit is full of antioxidants like beta-carotene that can protect your skin from sunburn?[40-42]

Did you know that pineapples contain bromelain, a powerful extract with anti-inflammatory and pain-relieving properties?[43-44]

Veggies are Vital

As tempting as it may be, we can't live on fruit alone. Vegetables, particularly leafy greens, are so important on a raw food diet.

The main reason for this is because fruits tend to be low in certain minerals like calcium, iron, and sodium. On the other hand, green vegetables like romaine, spinach, kale, and broccoli are much higher in these nutrients (see Table 5.1 below).

Table 5.1 Mineral Content of Fruits and Vegetables By Calories

Nutrients	Bananas, raw (100 kcals)	Peaches, raw (100 kcals)	Romaine, raw (100 kcals)	Spinach, raw (100 kcals)
Calcium	5.6 mg	15.4 mg	194.1 mg	430.4 mg
Copper (mg)	01. mg	0.2 mg	0.3 mg	0.6 mg
Iron (mg)	0.3 mg	0.6 mg	5.7 mg	11.8 mg
Magnesium (mg)	30.3 mg	23.1 mg	82.4 mg	343.5 mg
Manganese (mg)	0.3 mg	0.2 mg	0.9 mg	3.9 mg
Phosphorus (mg)	24.7 mg	51.3 mg	176.5 mg	231 mg
Potassium (mg)	402.2 mg	487.2 mg	1452.9 mg	2426.1 mg
Selenium (mcg)	1.1 mcg	0.3 mcg	2.4 mcg	4.3 mg
Sodium (mg)	1.1 mg	0 mg	47.1 mg	343.5 mg
Zinc (mg)	0.2 mg	0.4 mg	1.4 mg	2.3 mg

Source: *http://cronometer.com/*

Although not often regarded as such, greens are a great source of omega-3 fatty acids as well.* You just have to eat a lot of them, which isn't a problem since I know you'll be consuming tons of them on a healthy raw food diet!

Don't Load Up on Fat

I know I've said it a lot already, but that's because it's really important. If you want to truly thrive on raw foods, your fat intake needs to be low.

What exactly do I mean by low?

Ideally, you want your fat intake to come in at or a little below 10% of total calories.** This will help to ensure a high intake of fruits and vegetables (since you won't fill up on nuts and avocados), proper insulin sensitivity, and a healthy omega-6 to omega-3 ratio.***

To be clear, I mean 10% fat *overtime*. Having a day where you eat 20, 30, or even 60% fat is fine as long as your fat intake is low in the long-run.

Raw Food Formula for Success

If I were to illustrate the perfect raw food pyramid, it would look something like this…

---

* In 2012, I actually tested the fatty acid levels in my blood after consuming only fruit, greens, and omega-6 rich nuts and seeds (pistachios, Brazil nuts, sunflower seeds, and jungle peanuts) for several months. My results, including my omega-6 to omega-3 ratio (less than 3:1), were great. I even made a video showing these results, which you can see here: *http:// www.fitonraw.com/2012/09/my-raw-vegan-fatty-acid-blood-test-omega-3-epa-dha/*

** Some people may experience benefits with a slightly lower fat intake (around 5%), like better digestion and improved athletic performance. Others may experience improvements with a slightly higher fat intake (around 15%), like more supple skin and increased libido. It's also good to experiment to find out what works best for you!

*** If you want to consume more fat, say around 15% of total calories, it's best to focus on omega-3 rich sources like walnuts, chia seeds, and flax seeds. Otherwise, you may end up taking in too much omega-6 and throwing your fatty acid ratio out of whack.

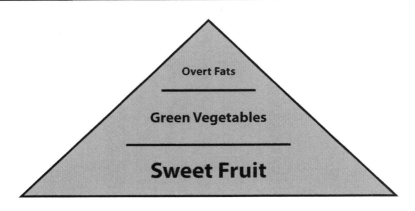

Fruit Comes First

On a healthy raw food diet, fruit is your fuel source.* The majority of your calories will come from sweet fruits like grapes, oranges, apples, cantaloupe, bananas, blueberries, mangoes, pears, papaya, watermelon, and peaches.**

To accomplish this, most (if not all) of your meals will contain fruit. Fruit for breakfast, fruit for lunch, and fruit for dinner followed by a large vegetable-based meal is a very common meal plan. However, if you don't need a ton of calories, you may find that having fruit for just breakfast and lunch does the trick.

Green Veggies Are Great, Too

To meet all of your mineral needs, you've got to get in plenty of greens. For most people, especially women who eat less calories overall, this means consuming *at least* one pound of green vegetables per day.*** This

---

* While foods like tomatoes, cucumber, zucchini, and bell pepper are technically fruits, their nutritional makeup is more similar to vegetables. They're also lower in calories like vegetables, which is why I do not include them at the base of the pyramid.

** While citrus fruits like oranges and grapefruit are certainly healthy foods, they are quite acidic and can wear away the enamel on your teeth. For this reason, it probably isn't a good idea to make them a staple in the diet. Personally, I tend to only eat these foods during the winter months when they're most sweet and least acidic. Even then, I do not eat them everyday for the entire season.

*** If you need a lot of calories (3,000+), you may not need as many veggies simply because you will be able to meet more of your mineral needs from all the fruit in your diet. How can you tell if you need more greens in your diet? I've found the following advice from Dr. Douglas Graham, author of *The 80/10/10 Diet*, to be very useful: If you crave salty or savory foods, you need more greens.[45] Getting yearly blood tests is a good idea as well.

will help make sure that you're getting plenty of calcium, iron, sodium, and other minerals that may be lacking on a fruit-only diet.

What exactly do I mean by greens? I mean tender leafy greens like romaine, spinach, iceberg, bib, and red leaf lettuce, but I also mean dark, tougher greens like kale, bok choy, swiss chard, and collard greens. Cruciferous vegetables like broccoli and cabbage can also be included.

That said, if you find the tougher greens like kale and broccoli too bitter or difficult to digest, you don't have to include them in your diet. As long as you eat plenty of the more tender greens and get in good variety throughout the year, you should take in plenty of minerals.*

Don't Forget Your Fats!

I know I've been pretty harsh on fats in this book. But that doesn't mean I think overt fats like avocados and nuts should be avoided. Quite the contrary!

I think these foods are very healthy and hold an important place, albeit a small one, in a raw food diet. For instance, sunflower seeds are full of vitamin E, macadamia nuts contain lots of manganese, and Brazil nuts are by far the best source of selenium.

And certain nuts and seeds like walnuts and flax seeds are excellent sources of omega-3 fatty acids. Just one ounce of flax seeds contains over six grams of this essential fat!

As great as these foods are, they are high in fat and do need to be limited. For most people, we're looking at one ounce of nuts/seeds or half an avocado per day. That will put you at about 10% if you eat around 2000 calories. If you eat more calories, feel free to up your overt fat intake a little bit.

---

* By variety, I don't mean you have to eat a different kind of vegetable every day through-out the week. Eating spinach and only spinach for a whole week or even several weeks isn't a problem as long as you're eating other green vegetables in sufficient quantities throughout the year.

How Many Calories Do I Need?

Since your caloric needs will depend upon several factors (age, height, gender, metabolism, activity level, etc.), I can't possibly tell you exactly how many calories you need. However, I can help you estimate for yourself how many you need.

If you know how many calories you eat on your current diet, then simply eat the same amount on a raw food diet. If you're used to eating 3000 calories, shoot for 3000 calories from fresh fruits and vegetables. You may find that you need more or less on raw, which is normal.

If you don't know how many calories you currently consume, here are some simple guidelines that should help.

For active women, a good starting place is 2000 calories per day.* You'll likely find that you need more or less than this, which is fine.** Simply adjust your meals accordingly.

For active men, 2500 calories per day is a good place to start.* Again, you may need more or less than this number.

To track your calories, I recommend CRON-O-Meter (_www. cronometer.com_). It's free, easy to use, and let's you set your own nutritional targets.

Sample Raw Meal Plans*

Now that you've seen the raw food formula for success, you may be wondering what all this looks like in practice. To help answer that question, here are seven sample days of low fat, high fruit, greens-filled raw eating.

---

* What if you're an _inactive_ man or woman? Then you may require less calories. But please, I urge you to adopt some sort of exercise routine, even if it's just walking around your neighborhood, as soon as you can. Being physically active is so important to your health and well-being. Stay tuned for chapter eight where I talk much more about the benefits of exercise, as well as the best forms of exercise for health and body composition.

** How do you know if you're eating too many or too few calories. If you're eating too many, you'll gain unwanted body fat. You may also feel bloated and uncomfortable after meals. If you're eating too few, you'll likely be hungry after meals (usually for sweet or starchy foods) and find it hard to maintain a healthy body weight.

Day 1

Breakfast

3 lbs papaya

Lunch

Banana, Orange, Spinach Smoothie
- 5 medium bananas
- 4 navel oranges
- 5 oz spinach (3 huge handfuls)
- water if needed

Blend.

Dinner

1) 1.5 lbs strawberries

2) Broccoli with Creamy Cashew Dip
- 1 lb fresh broccoli florets
- 1 oz raw cashews, soaked for at least one hour*
- juice from half of one small orange
- fresh or dried dill to taste
- water to blend

Blend the cashews, orange juice, dill, and water until smooth and creamy. Pour into a bowl and devour with the broccoli florets.

Calories

2034 calories
- 83.5% carbs
- 6.9% protein
- 9.6% fat

Day 2

Breakfast

Apples with Chocolatey Date Dip
- 4 medium apples
- 10 small dates, soaked for one hour if dry
- carob powder to taste
- water to blend

Blend the dates, carob, and water until smooth and creamy. Pour into a bowl, slice the apples, and dip away!

Lunch

2 lbs red grapes

Dinner

1) Chilly Citrus Smoothie
- 1 lb frozen pineapple
- 4 navel oranges

Peel the oranges and blend with the pineapple.

2) Romaine with Tomato Herb Dressing
- 1 lb romaine lettuce
- 1 cucumber
- 8 oz sugar snap peas
- 4 roma tomatoes
- 8 pieces sun-dried tomato, soaked for at least one hour
- basil to taste
- tarragon to taste
- parsley to taste
- water to blend

Chop the greens, slice the cucumber, and add to a large bowl with the peas. Pulse the fresh and dried tomatoes, herbs, and water in a blender until combined but still slightly chunky (be careful not to add too much water). Pour into the bowl and mix together.

Calories

2160 calories
- 92.1% carbs
- 5.2% protein
- 2.7% fat

Day 3

Breakfast

3 lbs peaches and one medium head iceberg lettuce

Lunch

2.5 lbs mangoes

Dinner

1) 1 lb watermelon

2) Kale and Avocado Salad
- 1 lb curly green kale
- 1 lb cherry or grape tomatoes
- 1/2 of one avocado
- 2 scallions
- juice from one small lime
- dulse to taste

De-stem and chop the kale into very small pieces and add to a large bowl. Halve the tomatoes, chop the scallions, and add to the bowl along with the scallions, and lime juice. Massage everything together for 3-5 minutes. Be sure to wear gloves if you have any cuts on your hands! Sprinkle as much dulse as you like on top.

Calories

1932 calories
- 82.1% carbs
- 7.6% protein
- 10.3% fat

Day 4

Breakfast

Mango Cherry Smoothie
- 2 lbs ataulfo mangoes
- 1 cup cherries, fresh or frozen
- water to blend

Blend.

Lunch

2 lbs figs and eight stalks of celery

Dinner

1) Savory Spinach Salad
- 16 oz baby spinach
- 1 cucumber
- 2 carrots
- 1 oz raw Brazil nuts, soaked for at least one hour
- juice from one lemon
- celery powder to taste*
- water to blend

Tear the spinach, slice the cucumber, peel and grate the carrots and add to a bowl. Blend the nuts, lemon juice, celery powder, and water until smooth and creamy. Pour over the greens, cucumber, and carrots, and mix together.

Calories

1986 calories

- 81% carbs
- 6.8% protein
- 12.3% fat

---

* To make your own celery powder, simply slice celery stalks into 1/2" slices and dry for several hours in a dehydrator. It's incredibly delicious and an excellent salt substitute.

Day 5

Breakfast

3 lbs cantaloupe

Lunch

Peach, Pineapple, Coconut Smoothie
- 1.5 lbs peaches, fresh or frozen
- 1 lb pineapple
- 1 cup coconut water

Blend.

Dinner

1) 2 lbs pears (any variety)

2) Romaine with Orange Date Dressing
- 16 oz romaine lettuce
- 6 Medjool dates
- juice from 2 oranges
- 1" piece of ginger
- celery powder to taste

Chop the romaine and place in a large bowl. Blend the dates, orange juice, ginger, and celery powder and combine with the greens.

Calories

2093 calories
- 91.3% carbs
- 5.3% protein
- 3.3% fat

	Day 6

Breakfast

Clementine & Kiwi Fruit Salad
- 2 lbs clementines
- 1 lb gold kiwi

Peel all the fruit and combine in a large bowl.

Lunch

Banana Blueberry Kale Smoothie
- 5 medium bananas
- 2 cups frozen wild blueberries
- 2 cups chopped dinosaur kale
- carob to taste

De-stem the kale and blend together with the fruit and carob. Use as much or as little water as you need to achieve the consistency that you like.

Dinner

1) Papaya Cauliflower Salad
- 16 oz red leaf lettuce
- 8 oz cauliflower
- 2 lbs papaya

Chop the lettuce, grate the cauliflower (or pulse in a food processor), and combine with the papaya flesh.

Calories

1953 calories
- 88.7% carbs
- 6.5% protein
- 4.8% fat

Day 7

Breakfast

Nectarine Berry Salad
- 2 lbs nectarines
- 1 lb plums
- 2 cups blueberries

Pit and chop the nectarines and plums and combine with the berries.

Lunch

6 medium bananas

Dinner

1) Collard Wraps with Nutty Pepper Sauce
- 2 bunches collard greens
- 2 large red bell pepper
- 2 cucumbers
- 3 carrots, peeled
- 2 oz walnut seeds
- 1 large orange bell pepper
- juice from one lemon
- cumin to taste
- water to blend

Blend the walnuts, orange pepper, lemon juice, cumin, and water until creamy and smooth. De-stem the collard greens and thinly slice the red pepper, cucumber, and carrot. Spread the sauce onto each collard leaf, top with some sliced veggies, wrap by folding the left and right side followed by the top and bottom, flip over, slice on the diagonal, and enjoy!

Calories

2215 calories

- 74.2% carbs
- 7.4% protein
- 18.5% fat**

---

* I've included a lot of variety in this menu simply to show you the many different fruits and vegetables available on a raw food diet. In reality, your weekly menu will likely be much more simple and be based upon what's in season in your area.

** It's generally recommended to consume overt fats later in the day after you've eaten all the fruit you care for. This is because fat digests more slowly than carbohydrates and some avocado or nuts may inhibit your digestion of sweet fruit and cause gas and bloating. I've personally tried switching my lunch and dinner meal (a big salad with avocado or nuts/seeds for lunch and fruit meal for dinner) and found that I get some abdominal pain and bloating in the evening when I do so. Of course, feel free to experiment to find what works best for you.

When And How Often Should I Eat?

Some people advocate eating five to six meals per day. Some say three is best. Others say two is where it's at.

Personally, I don't think it matters. If you prefer eating several smaller meals per day, fine. If you like eating two super large ones, that's also fine. It's whatever works for you.

That said, I do think it's important that you eat actual meals. No grazing all day, please. * Eating all day means sugar and acid on your teeth all day, which means abundant fuel for cavity-causing germs.

What About Late-Night Eating?

Many raw foodists recommend finishing eating at least 3 hours before bed. This will lead to deeper, more restful sleep because your body won't be preoccupied with digesting a meal. Also, you won't be up and down all night running to use the restroom!

While I personally find this guideline difficult to stick with because I prefer to eat a late breakfast and often have a snack after my evening meal, I do see the benefit. I find that I sleep more soundly and wake up less during the night to use the restroom when I finish eating about three hours before I go to sleep.

However, I get virtually the same benefits from finishing my meals one and a half to two hours before bedtime. Sometimes I have nights where I eat later, but even then I sleep very well.

For me, finishing food at least one hour before bedtime works very well. Play around with it and find what works for you!

---

* That said, it can be difficult to eat enough fruit in one meal at first and grazing can really help you get enough calories. As long as the goal is to eat actual meals, I think grazing is a very useful strategy when you're new to this diet.

Overnight or Overtime?

When I went raw, I made the mistake that most people make when attempting to adopt a new healthy habit: I tried to do everything at once. I did a lot of research and read a lot of books and blogs and really thought I could go 100% raw right then and there.

I was wrong.

There were just so many factors involved, factors that required personal experience rather than nosing through a book. Learning when fruit is ripe is a good example. Learning how many calories you need and how much fruit you must eat to meet those needs is an even better one.

To figure out these things, you simply have to DO the diet. And this presents a problem for someone like myself who tries to do it all at once. You're bound to eat unripe fruit, underestimate how much food you need, run out of ripe food in the house and make other newbie mistakes along the way.

Now for someone who transitions to raw instead of going 100% overnight, this isn't a problem at all. This person will have the chance to learn all the ins and outs of doing the diet correctly without the pressure of eating all raw.

This is the approach my Mom took when she decided to adopt a vegan diet.

Instead of cutting out all animal products right then and there, she changed her diet gradually. She started by eliminating foods that she knew she wouldn't really miss (like meat) and then gradually reduced the other foods that she knew would be a struggle to give up (like cheese and yogurt).

Most importantly, she put no time limit on her transition. She would simply make small improvements when she felt mentally ready to do so or when she no longer enjoyed a particular food as much.

As a result, her transition to a vegan diet was easy and stress-free.

So I definitely recommend a gradual transition to raw. I just think the overnight approach is far too difficult for many of us to accomplish and can lead to unhealthy yo-yo dieting.

That's It?!

I can hear it now...

What about iron? What about selenium? What about protein, omega-3s, and B12? Is it really possible to get enough of these and all other nutrients on a diet of fruits, vegetables, nuts, and seeds?

Yes, it most certainly is possible and I'll show you how in the next chapter.*

---

* Can't imagine eating three papaya, six bananas, or a pound of romaine *plus* salad fixins in a single sitting? Be sure to check out this book's companion video "Simple Tips for Raw Food Success" at: www.scienceofraw.com/success

CHAPTER 6
How to Avoid Nutritional Deficiencies With Raw Foods

As I mentioned in the introduction to this book and have hopefully proved in the preceding chapter, eating a 100% raw food diet does not guarantee nutritional adequacy. In fact, if you don't pay attention to the types and amounts of foods you're eating, it's very likely that you'll end up deficient in a nutrient or two.

Wait, don't leave! While going raw successfully isn't as easy as sitting down to a jar of tahini and a bowl of dehydrated flax crackers, it's still pretty darn simple.

In this fifth chapter, I'll show you how you can meet your nutritional needs for all essential micronutrients (vitamins and minerals like vitamin A, thiamin, folate, calcium, iron, and zinc) easily and enjoyably on a low fat raw vegan diet.

But first…

A Brief Note About These Guidelines

Unless stated otherwise, the guidelines in this chapter are based on those set by the World Health Organization (WHO), a non-profit branch of the United Nations.

Why did I choose WHO? Because many dietary guidelines—like America's Dietary Reference Intake (DRI)—cater to the average Westerner.

What does the average Westerner do? The average Westerner eats a high-fat, meat-rich, processed diet; consumes far too few fruits and vegetables; gets too little exercise and sunshine; and leads an otherwise unhealthy life.

On the other hand, WHO tends to set nutritional guidelines based upon various lifestyle factors—such as animal protein, salt, and phytate consumption—that affect nutrient absorption.

Let's take zinc as an example.

According to the Institute of Medicine, adult males need 9.4 mg of zinc per day.[1] According to WHO, adult males require anywhere from 4.2-14 mg of zinc every day depending upon the types of food that predominate in their diets. [2]

This is why I've decided to use the World Health Organization's guidelines as a basis for the following vitamin and mineral recommendations.[*]

The Essential Vitamins[**]

Vitamin A

Vitamin A is a fat-soluble vitamin necessary for proper vision, skin and bone health; gene expression; red blood cell production; and immune function. Carotenoids, vitamin A precursors, are awesome antioxidants that protect against free radical damage and cancer.

How Much Do We Need?
- Mean Requirement for Men: 300 mcg RAE/day[2]
- Mean Requirement for Women: 270 mcg RAE/day[2]

---

[*]   Please note that these recommendations are for healthy adult male and females only, not pregnant or lactating women, children, or adolescents.

[**]   Essential nutrients are those that can not be synthesized by the body and therefore must be consumed in the diet.

How Much Do Raw Foods Have?

You've probably heard that fruits and vegetables (particularly leafy greens) are excellent sources of vitamin A. That's not quite true. Fruits and vegetables are excellent sources of *carotenoids* like beta-carotene.

Carotenoids are provitamins that your body converts to retinol. Retinol, also known as preformed vitamin A, is only found in animal products.

Retinol activity equivalents (RAE) is the standard used to measure non-retinol vitamin A like beta-carotene found in plant foods. Dietary beta-carotene has an RAE ratio of 12:1, meaning you would have to consume 12 mcg of beta-carotene to get just 1 mcg of retinol. At 24:1, the RAE ratio for carotenoids like alpha-carotene and beta-cryptoxanthin is even poorer. [3]

Since you'll be taking in so much of these carotenoids on a fresh fruit and vegetable diet, these poor ratios aren't an issue. For instance, just 5 small papaya (338 calories) contain 2150.9 mcg of beta-carotene, 15.7 mcg of alpha-carotene, and 4623.6 mcg of beta-cryptoxanthin. When converted to RAE (i.e. 2150.9 ÷ 12 = 179.24), the total equals just over 370 mcg RAE.

So just by eating these papaya, a rather paltry meal calorie-wise, you'll EXCEED the mean requirement for vitamin A. Add some more fruit and lots of leafy greens and you'll easily get TONS of vitamin A.

Below is a sample 2000-calorie low fat raw vegan plan to give you some idea of the amount of vitamin A you'll consume on such a diet.

Table 6.1 Vitamin A Intake on a Low Fat Raw Diet

Meal	Food	Vitamin A (mcg RAE)
Breakfast	5 small papaya	372 mcg RAE
Lunch	7 medium bananas & 4 ounces (113 g) romaine	518.5 mcg RAE
Mid-Afternoon	1 pineapple	26.4 mcg RAE
Dinner	Salad of 12 ounces (340 g) spinach, 8 medium celery stalks, 1 cucumber, 4 medium tomatoes, juice from 1 lemon, 1 ounce (28 g) brazil nuts	1,887 mcg RAE
		2,804 mcg RAE (935-1004%)*

*Mean Requirement[2]

Thiamin (Vitamin B1)

Thiamin is a water-soluble B vitamin necessary for proper enzyme, nervous system, and muscular function, as well as carbohydrate metabolism.

How Much Do We Need?
- Recommended Nutrient Intake (RNI) for Men = 1.2 mg/day[2]
- Recommended Nutrient Intake (RNI) for Women = 1.1 mg/day[2]

How Much Do Raw Foods Have?

Virtually any combination of fresh fruit and vegetables as part of a healthy raw diet—assuming the diet is sufficient in calories and contains enough greens—will contain plenty of thiamin.

Below is a sample 2000-calorie low fat raw vegan plan to give you some idea of the amount of thiamin you'll consume on such a diet.

Table 6.2 Thiamin Intake on a Low Fat Raw Diet

Meal	Food	Thiamin (mg)
Breakfast	5 small papaya	0.2 mg
Lunch	7 medium bananas & 4 ounces (113 g) romaine	0.4 mg
Mid-Afternoon	1 pineapple	0.7 mg
Dinner	Salad of 12 ounces (340 g) spinach, 8 medium celery stalks, 1 cucumber, 4 medium tomatoes, juice from 1 lemon, 1 ounce (28 g) brazil nuts*	0.9 mg
		2.2 mg (183-200% RNI**)

*The brazil nuts only provide 0.2 mg of thiamin. Without them, you would still take in 2 mg, well above the RNI of 1.1 mg/day for women and 1.2 mg/day for men.
**Recommended Nutrient Intake[2]

Riboflavin (Vitamin B2)

Riboflavin is a water-soluble B vitamin necessary for carbohydrate metabolism, nervous system function, and red blood cell production. It's also an awesome antioxidant that protects against free radical damage and cancer.

How Much Do We Need?
- RNI for Men = 1.3 mg/day[2]
- RNI for Women = 1.1 mg/day[2]

How Much Do Raw Foods Have?

Virtually any combination of fresh fruit and vegetables as part of a healthy raw diet—assuming the diet is sufficient in calories and contains enough greens—will contain plenty of riboflavin.

Below is a sample 2000-calorie low fat raw vegan plan to give you some idea of the amount of riboflavin you'll consume on such a diet.

Table 6.3 Riboflavin Intake on a Low Fat Raw Diet

Meal	Food	Riboflavin (mg)
Breakfast	5 small papaya	0.2 mg
Lunch	7 medium bananas & 4 ounces (113 g) romaine	0.4 mg
Mid-Afternoon	1 pineapple	0.3 mg
Dinner	Salad of 12 ounces (340 g) spinach, 8 medium celery stalks, 1 cucumber, 4 medium tomatoes, juice from 1 lemon, 1 ounce (28 g) brazil nuts	1 mg
		1.9 mg (146-172% RNI*)

*Recommended Nutrient Intake[2]

Niacin (Vitamin B3)

Niacin is a water-soluble B vitamin necessary for healthy skin and digestion, carbohydrate metabolism, and nervous system function.

How Much Do We Need?
- RNI for Men = 16 mg/day[2]
- RNI for Women = 14 mg/day[2]

How Much Do Raw Foods Have?

Virtually any combination of fresh fruit and vegetables as part of a healthy raw diet—assuming the diet is sufficient in calories and contains enough greens—will contain plenty of niacin.

Below is a sample 2000-calorie low fat raw vegan plan to give you some idea of the amount of niacin you'll consume on such a diet.

Table 6.4 Niacin Intake on a Low Fat Raw Diet

Meal	Food	Niacin (mg)
Breakfast	5 small papaya	2.8 mg
Lunch	7 medium bananas & 4 ounces (113 g) romaine	5.9 mg
Mid-Afternoon	1 pineapple	4.5 mg
Dinner	Salad of 12 ounces (340 g) spinach, 8 medium celery stalks, 1 cucumber, 4 medium tomatoes, juice from 1 lemon, 1 ounce (28 g) brazil nuts	6.8 mg
		20 mg (125-143% RNI*)

*Recommended Nutrient Intake[2]

Pantothenic Acid (Vitamin B5)

Pantothenic acid is a water-soluble B vitamin necessary for brain development and function, hormone production, vitamin B12 absorption, and carbohydrate metabolism.

How Much Do We Need?
- RNI for Men = 5 mg/day[2]
- RNI for Women = 5 mg/day[2]

How Much Do Raw Foods Have?

Virtually any combination of fresh fruit and vegetables as part of a healthy raw diet—assuming the diet is sufficient in calories and contains enough greens—will contain plenty of pantothenic acid.

Below is a sample 2000-calorie low fat raw vegan plan to give you some idea of the amount of pantothenic acid you'll consume on such a diet.

Table 6.5 Pantothenic Acid Intake on a Low Fat Raw Diet

Meal	Food	Pantothenic Acid (mg)
Breakfast	5 small papaya	1.5 mg
Lunch	7 medium bananas & 4 ounces (113 g) romaine	3 mg
Mid-Afternoon	1 pineapple	1.9 mg
Dinner	Salad of 12 ounces (340 g) spinach, 8 medium celery stalks, 1 cucumber, 4 medium tomatoes, juice from 1 lemon, 1 ounce (28 g) brazil nuts	2.4 mg
		8.8 mg (176% RNI*)

*Recommended Nutrient Intake[2]

Vitamin B6 (Pyridoxine)

Pyridoxine is a water-soluble B vitamin necessary for growth, carbohydrate metabolism, red blood cell and hormone production, and proper digestion.

How Much Do We Need?
- RNI for Men = 1.3 mg per day[2]
- RNI for Women = 1.3 mg per day[2]

How Much Do Raw Foods Have?

Virtually any combination of fresh fruit and vegetables as part of a healthy raw diet—assuming the diet is sufficient in calories and contains enough greens—will contain plenty of pyridoxine.

Below is a sample 2000-calorie low fat raw vegan plan to give you some idea of the amount of pyridoxine you'll consume on such a diet.

Table 6.6 Pyridoxine Intake on a Low Fat Raw Diet

Meal	Food	Pyridoxine (mg)
Breakfast	5 small papaya	0.3 mg
Lunch	7 medium bananas & 4 ounces (113 g) romaine	3.1 mg
Mid-Afternoon	1 pineapple	1.0 mg
Dinner	Salad of 12 ounces (340 g) spinach, 8 medium celery stalks, 1 cucumber, 4 medium tomatoes, juice from 1 lemon, 1 ounce (28 g) brazil nuts	1.4 mg
		5.8 mg (446% RNI*)

*Recommended Nutrient Intake[2]

Folate (Vitamin B9)

Folate is a water-soluble B vitamin necessary for carbohydrate metabolism; red blood cell production; proper liver, brain, and nervous system function; as well as healthy hair and skin.

How Much Do We Need?
- RNI for Men = 400 mcg per day[2]
- RNI for Women = 400 mcg per day[2]

How Much Do Raw Foods Have?

Leafy greens like romaine and spinach are the best sources of this necessary nutrient, but other vegetables and fruit are good sources as well. Virtually any combination of fresh fruit and vegetables as part of a healthy raw diet—assuming the diet is sufficient in calories and contains enough greens—will contain plenty of folate.

Below is a sample 2000-calorie low fat raw vegan plan to give you some idea of the amount of folate you'll consume on such a diet.

Table 6.7 Folate Intake on a Low Fat Raw Diet

Meal	Food	Folate (mcg)
Breakfast	5 small papaya	290.4 mcg
Lunch	7 medium bananas & 4 ounces (113 g) romaine	318.9 mcg
Mid-Afternoon	1 pineapple	162.9 mcg
Dinner	Salad of 12 ounces (340 g) spinach, 8 medium celery stalks, 1 cucumber, 4 medium tomatoes, juice from 1 lemon, 1 ounce (28 g) brazil nuts	885.5 mcg
		1,657.7 mcg (414% RNI*)

*Recommended Nutrient Intake[2]

Vitamin B12 (Cobalamin)

Vitamin B12 is a water-soluble B vitamin necessary for carbohydrate metabolism, red blood cell and DNA production, and nervous system function.

How Much Do We Need?
- RNI for Men = 2.4 mcg/day[2]
- RNI for Women = 2.4 mcg/day[2]

How Much Do Raw Foods Have?

I won't say much about vitamin B12 here in this chapter other than the fact that a raw plant-based diet is not a reliable source of this necessary nutrient.

But don't worry! In the following chapter, I'll give you the full scoop on B12 and show you how easy it is to get enough on a low fat raw vegan diet.

Vitamin C (Ascorbate)

Vitamin C is a water-soluble vitamin necessary for collagen production, wound healing, and a healthy immune system. It's also an awesome antioxidant that protects against free radical damage and cancer.

How Much Do We Need?
- RNI for Men = 45 mg/day[2]
- RNI for Women = 45 mg/day[2]

How Much Do Raw Foods Have?

Everyone knows that fresh fruit and vegetables—remember, vitamin C is very sensitive to heat—are chock full of vitamin C. For example, just one cup of chopped red bell pepper contains almost 200 mg of this vital vitamin!

Below is a sample 2000-calorie low fat raw vegan plan to give you some idea of the amount of vitamin C you'll consume on such a diet.

Table 6.8 Vitamin C Intake on a Low Fat Raw Diet

Meal	Food	Vitamin C (mg)
Breakfast	5 small papaya	478.1 mg
Lunch	7 medium bananas & 4 ounces (113 g) romaine	76.4 mg
Mid-Afternoon	1 pineapple	432.6 mg
Dinner	Salad of 12 ounces (340 g) spinach, 8 medium celery stalks, 1 cucumber, 4 medium tomatoes, juice from 1 lemon, 1 ounce (28 g) brazil nuts	200 mg
		1,187.1 mg (2638% RNI*)

*Recommended Nutrient Intake[2]

Vitamin D

Vitamin D is a fat-soluble vitamin (i.e. your body can store it) necessary for bone health, immune system function, and cellular growth.

How Much Do We Need?
- RNI for Men = 5 mcg/day[2]
- RNI for Women = 5 mcg/day[2]

How Much Do Raw Foods Have?

It's called the sunshine vitamin for a reason, folks. The best source is not the food you eat, but skin exposure to the sun's rays.

I talk much more about getting enough of this vital vitamin in the following chapter, so stay tuned!

Vitamin E

Vitamin E is a fat-soluble vitamin necessary for proper immune function, red blood cell production, and gene expression. It's also an awesome antioxidant that protects against free radical damage and cancer.

How Much Do We Need?
- Total Polyunsaturated Fatty Acids (Omega-3 + Omega-6) x 0.4 = Vitamin E Requirement[2]

While the DRI for vitamin E is 15 mg per day for men and women, the truth is that vitamin E requirements are largely dependent upon consumption of polyunsaturated fats, particularly omega-6s.[2 & 4]

As mentioned in chapter two, omega-6 fatty acids (linoleic acid) cause oxidative damage. Antioxidants like vitamin E protect against this damage so the more linoleic acid you consume, the more vitamin E (as well as other antioxidants) you will require in your diet.5

So how much vitamin E would a raw vegan need? According to the 2004 WHO report "Vitamin and Mineral Requirements in Human Nutrition":

"It has been suggested that when the main PUFA [polyunsaturated fatty acid] in the diet is linoleic acid, a d-a-tocopherol-PUFA ratio of 0.4 (expressed as mg tocopherol [vitamin E] per g PUFA) is adequate for adult humans."[2]

On a healthy low fat raw vegan diet like the 2000-calorie plan shown below, total polyunsaturated fat consumption equals 8.8 grams, making the vitamin E requirement only 3.52 mg (8.8 g x 0.4). As you'll soon see, it's incredibly easy to meet and exceed this amount with raw foods.

How Much Do Raw Foods Have?

Below is a sample 2000-calorie low fat raw vegan plan to give you some idea of the amount of vitamin E you'll consume on such a diet.

Table 6.9 Vitamin E Intake on a Low Fat Raw Diet

Meal	Food	Vitamin E (mg)
Breakfast	5 small papaya	2.4 mg
Lunch	7 medium bananas & 4 ounces (113 g) romaine	0.9 mg
Mid-Afternoon	1 pineapple	0.2 mg
Dinner	Salad of 12 ounces (340 g) spinach, 8 medium celery stalks, 1 cucumber, 4 medium tomatoes, juice from 1 lemon, 1 ounce (28 g) brazil nuts	12.3 mg
		15.8 mg (449%*)

*This recommendation is based on the aforementioned PUFA to vitamin E ratio. The World Health Organization (WHO) has no official recommendation at this time due to insufficient evidence.[2]

Vitamin K

Vitamin K is a fat-soluble vitamin necessary for proper blood clotting and bone health.

How Much Do We Need?
- RNI for Men = 65 mcg per day[2]
- RNI for Women = 55 mcg per day[2]

How Much Do Raw Foods Have?

Fruits and vegetables, particularly leafy greens, are full of vitamin K. Just 8 ounces of romaine lettuce contains more than double the RNI for women!

Below is a sample 2000-calorie low fat raw vegan plan to give you some idea of the amount of vitamin K you'll consume on such a diet.

Table 6.10 Vitamin K Intake on a Low Fat Raw Diet

Meal	Food	Vitamin K (mcg)
Breakfast	5 small papaya	20.4 mcg
Lunch	7 medium bananas & 4 ounces (113 g) romaine	119.9 mcg
Mid-Afternoon	1 pineapple	6.3 mcg
Dinner	Salad of 12 ounces (340 g) spinach, 8 medium celery stalks, 1 cucumber, 4 medium tomatoes, juice from 1 lemon, 1 ounce (28 g) brazil nuts	1,824 mcg
		1,970.6 mcg (3031-3582% RNI)*

*Recommended Nutrient Intake[2]

The Essential Minerals[*]

Calcium

Calcium is a mineral necessary for bone, teeth, heart, and muscle health, as well as blood clotting.

How Much Do We Need?
- RNI for Men = 450 mg/day (based on low animal protein, low salt diet)[2]
- RNI for Women = 450 mcg/day (based on low animal protein, low salt diet)[2]

Americans consume more calcium than almost any other nation and yet the United States has one of the highest rates of osteoporotic hip fractures in the world. [6-7]

And Americans aren't alone. Other industrialized nations like England and Norway also have high rates of hip fractures and osteoporosis, much higher than developing countries in Asia and South Africa where calcium intake is significantly lower. [7]

The fact that Westerners consume so much bone-building calcium yet experience such high rates of hip fractures is known as the "calcium paradox".[2] And as with all paradoxes, no contradiction really exists. There is simply a lack or misunderstanding of information.

In the case of the calcium paradox, Western diets are high in animal protein and salt and low in fruits and vegetables. Both animal protein—including calcium-rich dairy—and salt force your body to excrete calcium, while fruits and vegetables actually prevent calcium excretion.[8-11, 12-13]

Other substances commonly consumed by Westerners that either increase calcium excretion or interfere with calcium absorption include alcohol, cigarettes, certain drugs like corticosteroids, caffeine, and grains.[14-15, 16-17, 18, 19-21, 22]

---

[*] Essential nutrients are those that can not be synthesized by the body and therefore must be consumed in the diet.

This is why calcium requirements for Westerners are typically set at 700-1000 mg per day. You have to consume that much to offset the calcium-reducing effects of your unhealthy meat, salt, alcohol, and drug-heavy diets.

But what if you're not consuming lots of animal products and salt? What if you eat a low fat raw vegan diet that's completely devoid of these substances yet full of fruits and vegetables? Would you still need 1000 mg of calcium on such a diet?

Nope.

According to the World Health Organization, someone consuming low amounts of animal protein and sodium would only need roughly 450 mg of calcium per day. Factors that improve absorption such as adequate vitamin D could reduce this amount even further.[2]

As I show below, it's ridiculously easy to meet and exceed this amount on a diet of fresh fruit, vegetables, nuts and seeds.

How Much Do Raw Foods Have?

Vegetables, particularly leafy greens, are excellent sources of calcium. The key is to consume enough of them.

Below is a sample 2000-calorie low fat raw vegan plan to give you some idea of the amount of calcium you'll consume on such a diet.

Table 6.11 Calcium Intake on a Low Fat Raw Diet

Meal	Food	Calcium (mg)
Breakfast	5 small papaya	157 mg
Lunch	7 medium bananas & 4 ounces (113 g) romaine	78.6 mg
Mid-Afternoon	1 pineapple	117.6 mg
Dinner	Salad of 12 ounces (340 g) spinach, 8 medium celery stalks, 1 cucumber, 4 medium tomatoes, juice from 1 lemon, 1 ounce (28 g) brazil nuts	610.3 mg
		963.5 mg (214% Recommendation*)

*This theoretical recommendation is based on a diet low in animal protein and salt. The recommended intake for those consuming a standard Western diet (approximately 60-80 grams of animal protein per day) is 1000 mg/day.[2]

Copper

Copper is a mineral necessary for red blood cell production, as well as healthy immune and nervous system functioning.

How Much Do We Need?

- RNI for Men (65 kg) = 1.35 mg/day[23]
- RNI for Women (55 kg) = 1.15 mg/day[23]

How Much Do Raw Foods Have?

You don't have to eat organs, oysters, or other animal products to get enough copper. A diet of fruit and greens will provide plenty of this necessary nutrient.

Below is a sample 2000-calorie low fat raw vegan plan to give you some idea of the amount of copper you'll consume on such a diet.

Table 6.12 Copper Intake on a Low Fat Raw Diet

Meal	Food	Copper (mg)
Breakfast	5 small papaya	0.4 mg
Lunch	7 medium bananas & 4 ounces (113 g) romaine	0.7 mg
Mid-Afternoon	1 pineapple	1.0 mg
Dinner	Salad of 12 ounces (340 g) spinach, 8 medium celery stalks, 1 cucumber, 4 medium tomatoes, juice from 1 lemon, 1 ounce (28 g) brazil nuts	1.4 mg
		3.5 mg (259-304% RNI)*

*Recommended Nutrient Intake[23]

Iron

Iron is a mineral necessary for red blood cell and energy production, as well as oxygen transportation and DNA synthesis.

How Much Do We Need?
- RNI for Men (75 kg) = 9.1-11.4 mg/day (based on 12-15% bio-availability)[2]
- RNI for Menstruating Women (62 kg) = 19.6-24.5 mg/day (based on 12-15% bioavailability)[2]

Like calcium, the amount of iron we need is largely dependent upon the foods we consume. A diet high in meat will have a relatively high absorption rate because meat contains heme iron, which is more easily absorbed than non-heme iron.

A diet high in grains and legumes, however will have a low absorption rate because these foods are comprised of non-heme iron AND, as I discussed in chapter three, they contain high amounts of phytates and other anti-nutrients that inhibit iron absorption.

So where does a low fat raw vegan diet fit in?

On the one hand, a low fat raw vegan diet is devoid of meat and the more easily absorbed heme iron. On the other hand, such a diet contains no grains (or very few grains) nor the high amounts of iron-inhibiting phytates that these foods contain. It's also free of other iron-inhibiting foods like dairy, coffee, tea, cocoa, and red wine.[2, 24-25, 26-27, 28]

Plus, a low fat raw vegan diet is very high in vitamin C, which has been shown to enhance iron absorption.[29-31] In fact, one study showed that ascorbic acid (vitamin C) was better at improving iron status than iron supplements![32]

In another study, anemic children given 100 mg of ascorbic acid twice a day showed a "significant improvement in Hb [haemoglobin] level as well as in red cell morphology".[33]

According to the World Health Organization, you should consume at least 25 mg of vitamin C at each meal.[2] As I've already shown, it's easy to get plenty of vitamin C on a low fat raw vegan diet. Just 12 ounces (340 g) of spinach, a great source of iron, also contains almost 100 mg of vitamin C!

Because a low fat, high fruit raw food diet is incredibly rich in vitamin C and low in iron-inhibiting foods, I believe it's safe to say that such a diet likely has a moderate to high iron bioavailability (12-15%).[*] According to WHO, this means that a menstruating woman weighing 62 kg (136 lbs) would need roughly 19.6-24.5 mg of iron per day, while a 75 kg (165 lb) male would need 9.1-11.4 mg per day.[2]

While meeting the 10 mg per day requirement for men is very easy to do on a low fat raw vegan diet, consuming 20-25 mg every day from food alone may pose a problem unless huge amounts of greens are consumed each day.

Which begs the question…

Do Women Really Need So Much Iron?

It's common knowledge that women need more iron than men simply due to blood lost during menstruation. According to the Institute of Medicine, the average menstruating woman requires 1.5 mg per day of iron.[**1]

However, it's also common knowledge (amongst non-meat eaters, anyway) that women who consume a vegan diet experience shorter, lighter periods than those who subsist on standard Western fare.[34-35]

Wouldn't it follow that women who bleed less need less iron?

That's certainly been my experience. Prior to going raw, I was anemic on both a standard Western diet as well as a grains-heavy vegan diet. Today I average only 15-20 mg of non-heme iron per day from fruits, vegetables, nuts and seeds yet I'm no longer anemic. My blood tests

---

[*]   I believe that it is very important to get blood work done regularly to verify that you are getting in enough iron, especially if you are menstruating.

[**]   Non-menstruating women lose only 0.9 to 1.02 mg/day and therefore require less iron in their diet.

taken in both June 2011 and 2012 showed my ferritin and iron stores within the normal ranges.*

Even still, 1.5 mg/day (the amount required by menstruating women) is not much.

Let's say you consume just 15 mg of iron per day from fresh fruits and vegetables. An assumed bioavailability of 15% would mean that your body would absorb 2.25 mg of iron per day. A lower bioavailability of 12% would mean 1.8 mg of iron per day would be absorbed, which is still higher than the 1.5 mg requirement.

The Problem with Animal Iron

As I already mentioned, animal products contain heme iron and plant foods contain non-heme iron. Heme iron is more bioavailable, meaning that it is more easily absorbed by your body.

So even though 3 ounces of ground beef and 10 ounces of broccoli contain the same amount of iron (2 mg), you would have to eat more of the broccoli to utilize the same amount of iron that you would absorb from the beef.

While this may sound bad, it's actually a good thing since excess heme iron is bad for the body. For one, iron is a pro-oxidant that causes oxidative stress and DNA damage.[36-37] Excess iron has also been linked to all sorts of health concerns, including heart disease, heart attacks, colon cancer, and even breast cancer.[38,39,40,37]

On a low fat raw vegan diet that contains only plant-foods, it's virtually impossible to take in too much iron.

How Much Do Raw Foods Have?

Most fruits are pretty low in iron, but leafy greens and other vegetables are excellent sources. The fact that these foods also contain vitamin C makes them even better sources of this magnificent mineral.

* The reference ranges for ferritin and iron (according to my lab report) are 10-291 ng/ml and 50-170 ug/dL, respectively. In 2011, my ferritin levels were 11 ng/ml and my iron 75 ug/ dL. In 2012, my ferritin levels were 13 ng/ml.

Below is a sample 2000-calorie low fat raw vegan plan to give you some idea of the amount of iron you'll consume on such a diet.

Table 6.13 Iron Intake on a Low Fat Raw Diet

Meal	Food	Iron (mg)
Breakfast	5 small papaya	2.0 mg
Lunch	7 medium bananas & 4 ounces (113 g) romaine	3.2 mg
Mid-Afternoon	1 pineapple	2.6 mg
Dinner	Salad of 12 ounces (340 g) spinach, 8 medium celery stalks, 1 cucumber, 4 medium tomatoes, juice from 1 lemon, 1 ounce (28 g) brazil nuts*	12.6 mg
		20.4 mg (104% RNI for women**, 224% RNI for men**)***

*This high-iron meal also contains 200 mg of vitamin C which will likely increase iron absorption significantly.
**Based on 15% bioavailability[2]
***Recommended Nutrient Intake[2]

Magnesium

Magnesium is a mineral necessary for bone and teeth health, muscle and nerve function, energy production, and protein synthesis.

How Much Do We Need?
- RNI for Men = 260 mg/day[2]
- RNI for Women = 220 mg/day[2]

How Much Do Raw Foods Have?

Leafy greens are full of magnesium and many fruits are great sources as well.

Below is a sample 2000-calorie low fat raw vegan plan to give you some idea of the amount of magnesium you'll consume on such a diet.

Table 6.14 Magnesium Intake on a Low Fat Raw Diet

Meal	Food	Magnesium (mg)
Breakfast	5 small papaya	164.8 mg
Lunch	7 medium bananas & 4 ounces (113 g) romaine	238.8 mg
Mid-Afternoon	1 pineapple	108.6 mg
Dinner	Salad of 12 ounces (340 g) spinach, 8 medium celery stalks, 1 cucumber, 4 medium tomatoes, juice from 1 lemon, 1 ounce (28 g) brazil nuts	506.5 mg
		1,018.7 mg (463% RNI for women, 392% RNI for men)*

*Recommended Nutrient Intake[2]

Manganese

Manganese is a mineral necessary for bone health, blood clotting, carbohydrate metabolism, and blood sugar regulation.

How Much Do We Need?
- 2-5 mg/day as adequate*

How Much Do Raw Foods Have?

Plenty. Just one cup of pineapple has 1.5 milligrams of this magnificent mineral.

Below is a sample 2000-calorie low fat raw vegan plan to give you some idea of the amount of manganese you'll consume on such a diet.

---

* More research on manganese requirements is needed so this recommendation is tentative.[23]

Table 6.15 Manganese Intake on a Low Fat Raw Diet

Meal	Food	Manganese (mg)
Breakfast	5 small papaya	0.3 mg
Lunch	7 medium bananas & 4 ounces (113 g) romaine	2.4 mg
Mid-Afternoon	1 pineapple	8.4 mg
Dinner	Salad of 12 ounces (340 g) spinach, 8 medium celery stalks, 1 cucumber, 4 medium tomatoes, juice from 1 lemon, 1 ounce (28 g) brazil nuts	4.4 mg
		15.5 mg (310-775%)*

* Tentative adequate intake. More research on manganese requirements is needed.[23]

Phosphorus

Phosphorus is a mineral necessary for bone and teeth health, carbohydrate metabolism, protein synthesis, and DNA and RNA production.

How Much Do We Need?
- DRI for Men = 700 mg/day*
- DRI for Women = 700 mg/day*

How Much Do Raw Foods Have?

While protein-rich foods like meat and dairy are typically thought of as the best sources of phosphorus, sufficient amounts of fruits and veggies will provide plenty of this magnificent mineral.

Plus, a healthy raw food diet has an ideal calcium to phosphorus ratio of about 1 to 1. Your typical meat and grain-rich Western diet contains too much phosphorus and not enough calcium, which can negatively affect bone health.[42]

Below is a sample 2000-calorie low fat raw vegan plan to give you some idea of the amount of phosphorus you'll consume on such a diet.

* No WHO recommendation is available for phosphorus so I have instead referred to the latest Dietary Reference Intake (DRI).[41]

125

Table 6.16 Phosphorus Intake on a Low Fat Raw Diet

Meal	Food	Phosphorus (mg)
Breakfast	5 small papaya	78.5 mg
Lunch	7 medium bananas & 4 ounces (113 g) romaine	215.6 mg
Mid-Afternoon	1 pineapple	72.4 mg
Dinner	Salad of 12 ounces (340 g) spinach, 8 medium celery stalks, 1 cucumber, 4 medium tomatoes, juice from 1 lemon, 1 ounce (28 g) brazil nuts	643 mg
		1,009.5 mg (144% RDA)*

*Recommended Daily Allowance (RDA)[41]

Potassium

Potassium is a mineral necessary for heart, muscular, and digestive function; carbohydrate metabolism; and protein synthesis.

How Much Do We Need?
- Adequate Intake (AI) for Men = 4.7 mg/day*
- Adequate Intake (AI) for Women = 4.7 mg/day*

How Much Do Raw Foods Have?

Fruits and vegetables are chock full of potassium. Even if you don't eat bananas (which aren't the highest source of potassium, anyway), you'll still get tons of this magnificent mineral.

Below is a sample 2000-calorie low fat raw vegan plan to give you some idea of the amount of potassium you'll consume on such a diet.

---

* No WHO recommendation for phosphorus is available so I have instead referred to the latest Dietary Reference Intake (DRI).[43]

Table 6.17 Potassium Intake on a Low Fat Raw Diet

Meal	Food	Potassium (mg)
Breakfast	5 small papaya	1,428.7 mg
Lunch	7 medium bananas & 4 ounces (113 g) romaine	3,236.2 mg
Mid-Afternoon	1 pineapple	986.4 mg
Dinner	Salad of 12 ounces (340 g) spinach, 8 medium celery stalks, 1 cucumber, 4 medium tomatoes, juice from 1 lemon, 1 ounce (28 g) brazil nuts	4,573.9 mg
		10,225.2 mg (218% AI)*

*Adequate Intake (AI)[43]

Selenium

Selenium is a mineral necessary for healthy immune function and is also an awesome antioxidant that protects against free radical damage and cancer.

How Much Do We Need?
- RNI for Men = 34 mg/day[2]
- RNI for Women = 26 mg/day[2]

How Much Do Raw Foods Have?

Most fruits and vegetables are rather low in selenium, but brazil nuts are an excellent source with incredible bioavailability of 90% or more.[2]

Below is a sample 2000-calorie low fat raw vegan plan (including brazil nuts) to give you some idea of the amount of selenium you'll consume on such a diet.

Table 6.18 Selenium Intake on a Low Fat Raw Diet

Meal	Food	Selenium (mcg)
Breakfast	5 small papaya	4.7 mcg
Lunch	7 medium bananas & 4 ounces (113 g) romaine	8.8 mcg
Mid-Afternoon	1 pineapple	0.9 mcg
Dinner	Salad of 12 ounces (340 g) spinach, 8 medium celery stalks, 1 cucumber, 4 medium tomatoes, juice from 1 lemon, 1 ounce (28 g) brazil nuts*	549.1 mcg
		563.5 mcg (1657-2167% RNI)**

*Minus the brazil nuts, this plan contains 20 mcg of selenium.
**Recommended Nutrient Intake[2]

Sodium

Sodium is a mineral necessary for blood volume and blood pressure maintenance, as well as proper brain, nerve, and muscular function.

How Much Do We Need?
- **Safe minimum = 500 mg/day[43-44]**

While it's fairly easy to consume 500 mg or more of sodium on a low fat raw food diet, I don't think this is necessary for most people.

Here's why:

First, hyponatremia—a condition of low sodium in the blood that can lead to nausea, vomiting, hallucinations, convulsions, coma, and even death—is very rare. It is typically only seen in endurance athletes, hospitalized elderly patients, and those taking diuretics.[43, 45-46]

In fact, studies have shown that hyponatremia does not occur in people consuming low-sodium diets (150-230 grams per day).[43]

The rarity of low serum sodium makes perfect sense. At no more than 460-920 mg/day, humans have evolved eating low amounts of sodium and our bodies have adapted to these intakes.[44]

Second, there are several examples of societies consuming much less sodium than this.[47] For instance, the Yanomamo of Brazil take in only 23 mg/day on average.[44] Not only have these societies shown almost no signs of hypertension, there has been no evidence of hyponatremia either.

Third, the Institute of Medicine admits that when "substantial sweating" is absent, average sodium loss is less than 180 mg of sodium per day, even amongst those living in tropical climates.[43]

In addition, it has been proven that once the body becomes acclimatized to increased sweating (which can take only a matter of days), there is a reduction in the amount of sodium lost via sweat.[43] In other words, your body has the amazing ability to adapt to excessive sweating by reducing the amount of sodium you excrete when you physically exert yourself.

Fourth, the 500 milligram minimum established in the latest RDA is for sodium chloride (salt), not just sodium.[43]

Chloride is found in all plant foods, particularly tomatoes, celery, kale, and kelp. And just like sodium, chloride deficiency (hypochloremia) is rare, even amongst people on low-salt diets.[43]

Finally, I consumed very low amounts of sodium (150 mg/day on average) for over two years. I never developed any symptoms of hyponatremia.

In conclusion, there is simply no evidence that the average moderately active adult needs 500 milligrams of sodium per day, much less 1500 milligrams.

It's much more likely that we need only 300 mg (or even less), which is personally the number that I aim for.

All that said, it's fairly easy to consume 500 milligrams or more of sodium every day on nothing but raw vegan foods, as long as you include sodium-rich sources in your diet.

How Much Do Raw Foods Have?

A diet of fruit and greens can be very low in sodium (~150 mg) so it's important to include some sodium-rich foods on a regular basis, especially if you are very active and/or live in a hot climate. (I talk more about this later on in the chapter.

Below is a sample 2000-calorie low fat raw vegan plan (with some sodium-rich sources) to give you some idea of the amount of sodium you'll consume on such a diet.

Table 6.19 Sodium Intake on a Low Fat Raw Diet

Meal	Food	Sodium (mg)
Breakfast	5 small papaya	62.8 mg
Lunch	7 medium bananas & 4 ounces (113 g) romaine	17.3 mg
Mid-Afternoon	1 pineapple	9 mg
Dinner	Salad of 12 ounces (340 g) spinach, 8 medium celery stalks, 1 cucumber, 4 medium tomatoes, juice from 1 lemon, 1 ounce (28 g) brazil nuts	556.6 mg
		645.7 mg (129%)*

*Safe minimum[44]

Zinc

Zinc is a mineral necessary for a healthy immune system; cell production, growth, and repair; and wound healing.

How Much Do We Need?
- RNI for Men = 7 mg/day (moderate bioavailability)[*2]
- RNI for Women = 4.9 mg/day (moderate bioavailability)[*2]

* WHO considers a vegan diet that is not based on cereal grains (like a low fat raw vegan diet) to be moderately bioavailable (30% absorption rate).[2]

How Much Do Raw Foods Have?

You don't have to eat calf's liver, venison, or crimini mushrooms to get enough zinc. A raw food diet sufficient in fruit and leafy greens will provide plenty of this magnificent mineral.

Below is a sample 2000-calorie low fat raw vegan plan to give you some idea of the amount of zinc you'll consume on such a diet.

Table 6.20 Zinc Intake on a Low Fat Raw Diet

Meal	Food	Zinc (mg)
Breakfast	5 small papaya	0.6 mg
Lunch	7 medium bananas & 4 ounces (113 g) romaine	1.5 mg
Mid-Afternoon	1 pineapple	1.1 mg
Dinner	Salad of 12 ounces (340 g) spinach, 8 medium celery stalks, 1 cucumber, 4 medium tomatoes, juice from 1 lemon, 1 ounce (28 g) brazil nuts	4.8 mg
		8 mg (163% RNI for women, 114% RNI for men)*

*Recommended Nutrient Intake[2]

Other Necessary Nutrients

Biotin, Chromium, Iodine, and Molybdenum

I neglected to mention the four essential nutrients biotin, chromium, iodine, and molybdenum not because they are unimportant, but because the data we have regarding the amounts present in various foods (as well as the amounts we need for good health) is either inconsistent or unavailable.[2 & 23]

In any event, this isn't a concern. A healthy low fat raw food diet should provide at least some of these nutrients while a multivitamin/multimineral supplement will cover the rest. (Please see the following chapter for more info on supplementation.)

Essential Amino Acids

Amino acids are the building blocks of protein and, contrary to popular opinion, you don't need to eat meat to get enough. All plant foods contain all essential amino acids in varying amounts, which is why it's important to include a good variety of fruits and vegetables in your diet.

Even a low fat raw vegan diet that's quite low in protein can provide plenty of the essential amino acids your body needs, as I show in the following table.

Table 6.21 Essential Amino Acids on a Low Fat Raw Vegan Diet

Essential Amino Acids	mg/kg per day	mg/54 kg (119 lbs) per day	mg from 2000 kcal sample raw diet*
Histidine	10 mg	540 mg	1,300 mg (241%)
Isoleucine	20 mg	1,080 mg	1,400 mg (130%)
Leucine	39 mg	2,106 mg	2,400 mg (114%)
Lysine	30 mg	1,620 mg	2,000 mg (123%)
Methionine + Cysteine	15 mg	810 mg	1,200 mg (148%)
Methionine	10 mg	–	–
Cysteine	4 mg	–	–
Phenylalanine + Tyrosine	25 mg	1,350 mg	2,500 mg (185%)
Threonine	15 mg	810 mg	1,300 mg (160%)
Tryptophan	4 mg	216 mg	400 mg (185%)
Valine	26 mg	1,404 mg	1,700 mg (121%)
Total Essential Amino Acids	184 mg	10,746 mg	14,200 mg (132%)

Source: Protein and Amino Acid Requirements in Human Nutrition[48]
*This is the same sample low fat raw food diet used throughout this chapter.

If you follow my raw food formula for success—lots of fruit, lots of green, limited amounts of fat—you should have no problem meeting your protein needs.

What About Toxicity?

You probably noticed that the sample low fat raw vegan food plan I used in this chapter provides more than the RNI for several nutrients. For instance, vitamin A is over 9 times the RNI while vitamin K is over 30 times the RNI!

Don't worry, this isn't a problem.

In the case of vitamin A, it's important to distinguish between preformed vitamin A (from animal products) and carotenoids like beta-carotene (from plants).

As I already mentioned, high intakes of preformed vitamin A found in animal foods have been linked to a reduction in bone mineral density and increased risk for osteoporosis and hip fractures.49 Beta-carotene and other carotenoids have never been associated with poor bone health.[1]

In fact, the Tolerable Upper Intake Level (UL) for vitamin A set by the Institute of Medicine pertains only to preformed vitamin A. There is no upper limit for plant-based vitamin A.[1]

In other words, it's virtually impossible to consume too much vitamin A on a low fat raw vegan diet.

In the case of vitamin K, "no adverse effects associated with vitamin K consumption from food or supplements have been reported in humans or animals."[1]

And it's the same for most other vitamins and minerals. Either no adverse effects have been reported or adverse effects have only resulted from large supplemental doses and/or high amounts of animal products in the diet.[1, 4, 41, 43, 50-51]

However, there are a few exceptions.

Folate

Folate has a UL of 1,000 mg/day from both supplements AND food, even though "no adverse effects have been associated with the consumption of the amounts of folate normally found in fortified foods."[50]

This is because some studies (but not all) have found that high amounts of folate may aggravate vitamin B12 deficiency and many people (particularly the elderly) are deficient in B12.[52-54]

For those of us who aren't B12 deficient—and you won't be, if you follow the advice offered in the next chapter—there's nothing to worry about with regard to a diet high in folate. In fact, the same researchers who found that excess folate can worsen B12 deficiency also found that a high serum folate was associated with "protection against cognitive impairment" in those with good B12 status.[54]

Manganese

Manganese has a UL of 11 mg/day for both food and supplements because of the devastating neurological effects seen in those exposed to manganese dust.[1]

While a plant-based diet can easily exceed this limit, manganese toxicity from food has never been reported and there is "presently no evidence that the consumption of a manganese-rich plant-based diet results in manganese toxicity."[1 & 55]

Selenium

The UL for selenium is 400 micrograms per day from both supplements AND food.[4] As I already mentioned, brazil nuts are an excellent source of selenium, with just one ounce containing 146 mcg ABOVE the daily limit!

Because of this, I recommend limiting your brazil nut consumption to no more than a few ounces per week.

Micronutrient Counting and Variety

Meeting all of your nutritional needs on a daily basis is unnecessary. There will likely be days when you are a little low in this or that nutrient. As long as you are eating a varied diet and getting the proper amount of nutrients overtime, this isn't an issue.

To be clear, eating a varied diet doesn't mean eating different foods for every meal, every day, every week, or even every month. Eating a varied diet means eating a variety of fruits, vegetables, nuts and seeds *throughout the year*. An easy way to accomplish this is to eat with the seasons.

For instance, let's say that it's winter and you've been eating lots of winter fruits like oranges, tangerines, dates, papaya, and broccoli. Then spring roles around and you now have access to a whole host of different fruits and vegetables like strawberries, Ataulfo mangoes, fennel, and peas.

A few months later, you're dining on summer produce like peaches, more mangoes, blueberries, melons, and zucchini. Once autumn hits, you'll have persimmons, grapes, apples, pears, and kale. By the end of the year, you will have eaten a whole host of fruits and vegetables.

To drive my point home, check out some of the different fruits and vegetables available in my ordinary supermarket (not Whole Foods or another speciality shop) throughout the year:

- Apples (Braeburn)
- Apples (Fuji)
- Apples (Gala)
- Apples (Golden, organic and conventional)
- Apples (Green, organic and conventional)
- Apples (Honey Crisp)
- Apples (Macintosh)
- Apples (Red Delicious, organic and conventional)
- Apples (Pink Lady)
- Bananas (organic and conventional)
- Bell pepper (organic and conventional)
- Bib lettuce (aka Boston or Butter lettuce)
- Blackberries
- Blueberries
- Bok choy
- Broccoli (conventional and organic)
- Cantaloupe (aka musk melon)
- Carrots (organic and conventional)
- Carrots (baby, organic and conventional)
- Celery (organic and conventional)

- Clementines
- Collard greens
- Concord grapes
- Coconut (mature)
- Cucumber (organic and conventional)
- Endive
- Fennel
- Florida avocado
- Grapes (black)
- Grapes (red, organic and conventional)
- Grapes (green, organic and conventional)
- Hass avocado (organic and conventional)
- Honeydew
- Iceberg lettuce (organic and conventional)
- Kale
- Kale (baby, organic)
- Kiwi (organic and conventional)
- Leaf lettuce (red)
- Leaf lettuce (green)
- Lemons
- Limes
- Oranges (Cara Cara)
- Oranges (Navel)
- Oranges (Valencia, aka juicing)
- Mixed greens (organic)
- Nectarines
- Papaya
- Peaches
- Pears (Asian)
- Pears (Bartlett)
- Pineapple
- Plantains
- Raddichio
- Raspberries
- Romaine lettuce (organic and conventional)
- Romaine (baby, organic)
- Spinach
- Spinach (baby, organic)
- Starfruit

- Strawberries
- Tangerines
- Tomatoes (beefsteak)
- Tomatoes (campari)
- Tomatoes (cherry, conventional and organic)
- Tomatoes (grape, conventional and organic)
- Tomatoes (on-the-vine, conventional and organic)
- Tomatoes (roma)
- Yellow squash
- Zucchini (organic and conventional)

Just by eating enough fruit to fulfill your caloric needs, getting in your greens, and eating a variety of fruits and vegetables throughout the year, you can easily meet all of your nutritional needs on a raw food diet.

Well, *most* of your needs...but I'll save that for the next chapter.

Avoid Nutrients for Nutrients Sake

The problem with nutrient-by-nutrient science...is that it takes the nutrient out of context of the food, the food out of context of the diet, and the diet out of context of the lifestyle. Marion Nestle, In Defense of Food by Michael Pollan

While ensuring that your diet contains an adequate supply of nutrients is incredibly important, choosing foods based solely on their concentration of one or two nutrients is not a good idea. Being high in this or that vitamin or mineral is not enough to qualify a food as health-promoting.

Let's pretend your diet is lacking in omega-3s. You learn that salmon is a good source of this fatty acid, but is salmon really a healthy food?

You already know from chapter one that the answer is no. Salmon is high in fat and cholesterol, contains no fiber, and is often contaminated with dangerous substances like PCBs.

English walnuts would be a much better choice for increasing your omega-3 intake. Not only are they an excellent source of this nutrient—just one ounce containing over 2.5 grams—but they're also rich in manganese and copper and low in cholesterol.

Now let's say you believe your diet is lacking sodium. The obvious choice would be salt, since it's the most concentrated source of this mineral. One teeny tiny teaspoon contains well over 2.5 grams of sodium, but is salt really a healthy food?

Not really. Salt is 99% sodium chloride and 1% trace minerals. Sure, you can buy speciality salts that are less processed, but the difference is minor. Himalayan sea salt is 95-98% sodium chloride and Celtic roughly 84%.

Celery is a much better choice for upping the sodium in your diet. Not only is it rich in sodium, celery is full of other important nutrients like fiber, vitamin A, folate, potassium, and manganese.

Listen to Your Body

While the guidelines in this chapter are meant to help you meet all of your nutrient requirements and thrive on a raw food diet, they are generalizations. Everyone is different.

Take me, for instance. Whether it's the dog days of summer and I'm sweating it out on the tennis courts or it's the middle of winter and I'm cozying up by the fire, 300 mg of sodium just doesn't cut it.

When I average this amount several days in a row, I start to want other foods after my nightly salad. Even though I'm full, I want more food. Inevitably, I eat more fruit (usually tomatoes or some other juicy fruit) until my belly is full to bursting.

This is a clear example of getting enough calories without getting enough nutrients.

However, when I average about 400-600 mg, this problem goes away. I feel satisfied after my meals, without the need to stuff myself silly. And it's a very easy fix. Just a few stalks of celery or a lovely meal of cantaloupe does the trick.

Why do I need so much sodium even when I'm, theoretically, not excreting very much? Who knows? Perhaps I'm just more active than I think and eliminate more than I think I do.

In any event, it may not be sodium at all. It may be some other nutrient that my body needs and that the celery, coconut water, spinach and cantaloupe provide.

My point is that the reason really doesn't matter. By listening to my body, I was able to notice the problem. By applying reason to that problem (i.e. checking my nutritional intake via CRON-O-Meter), I was able to identify that problem and implement the solution.

And chances are that you're just like me. Perhaps you need more selenium. Perhaps you need more zinc. Perhaps you burn crazy amounts of calories due to a speedy metabolism and/or poor absorption and get to eat more food altogether.

Lucky you!

By listening to your body, you'll be able to discern your own personal needs and make a low fat, high fruit raw vegan diet work best for you.

Fruit and Greens Are Your Friends

I hope I've shown you how easy and enjoyable it is to eat raw the right way. With few exceptions, your nutritional needs will be met by simply eating enough calories from fruit and getting in your greens.

You're wondering about those "few exceptions," aren't you? Good, because I'm getting to them right now.

CHAPTER 7
What About Supplements?*

When I first went raw in 2007 and for quite some time after, I didn't believe in supplementation. I thought as long as you were eating a healthy diet of fruits, vegetables, and limited amounts of nuts and seeds—and also paying adequate attention to other health factors such as sleep, sunshine, and exercise—you wouldn't need to supplement.

Then in 2011, I came upon long-term raw vegan Don Bennett's website (*www.health101.org*) and everything changed...

Mellon Belly: Normal or a Cause for Concern?

There's a terrible, horrible condition running rampant through the low fat, high fruit raw vegan community. It's called melon belly (I believe the scientific name is *melonus bellicificus*) and it's so scary, so terrifying, that it just might turn you off of raw foods for good!

Okay, I may be exaggerating a little bit.

Melon belly, as it's known amongst raw foodies, simply refers to stomach pain that occurs during and after eating melons like cantaloupe, honeydew, or watermelon. Some people experience it eating other fruits like grapes and apples and some also have pain in the back and/or chest. The pain is typically mild, although it can be quite intense, and usually disappears within 15-30 minutes.[1]

---

* This chapter is dedicated to low fat raw vegan Don Bennett. Without his knowledge and experience, I may never have taken a second look at supplements and learned how important they can be as part of a healthy raw food diet. Thanks, Don!

Most low fat raw vegans don't make a big deal out of melon belly and think it's the result of eating too much food in one sitting. Melons are water-rich, low-calorie fruits so this is fairly easy to do.

Like many low fat raw vegans, I have struggled with melon belly in the past. Watermelon wasn't too bad, but grapes and apples gave me quite a bit of abdominal pain. It was rare for me to eat more than a pound of grapes or a few apples in one sitting without pain.

I definitely wasn't overeating on just one pound of grapes and a few apples. What was *really* going on?

At first I thought it might be a reaction to pesticide residue on the fruit, since I was eating conventionally grown grapes and apples. So I tried organic instead, but got the same painful results.

Then I tried eating very very slowly, chewing as much as possible and waiting at least 30 seconds between bites. Again, same results.

Finally, I came across an article on melon belly by long-term raw vegan Don Bennett. Don writes:

> **A possible reason for discomfort or pain after eating a mono-meal of sweet fruit has been shown to be a lack of sufficient chromium in the diet. Chromium is known to enhance the action of insulin, which is a hormone critical to the metabolism and storage of carbohydrate, fat, and protein in the body.**[2]

Huh?

As I said before, I was of the opinion that supplementation was unnecessary. I was eating a healthy low fat raw vegan diet so why would I have a deficiency?

But Don's article was persuasive so I did as he advised. I bought some chromium supplements (chromium picolinate) from my local Whole Foods Market and took one dose of 200 mcg every day for two weeks.

After a few days of supplementation, I tested the theory with some grapes. I ate one pound of grapes with no pain. So far so good. Then I ate a few more grapes. Still no pain.

I ended up eating two full pounds of grapes without any pain!

Just to be sure, I stopped taking the chromium after 14 days. A few days later, my painful symptoms started to come back!

The evidence was crystal clear. My melon belly wasn't due to overeating, eating too fast, or eating conventionally-grown produce. It was due to a chromium deficiency.

This got me thinking...

If the fruits and vegetables I'm eating are very likely deficient in chromium, what other nutrients might my diet be lacking?

Vitamin B12: Ditch the Dogma

Like many raw foodists, I used to believe that getting enough B12 simply meant improving my absorption rate by avoiding things like drugs, alcohol, and processed foods and eating lots of organic fruits and vegetables. I thought supplementation was unnecessary in most cases.

I now see this viewpoint for what it really was: wishful thinking. *Dangerous* wishful thinking, in fact, since B12 deficiency can cause serious neurological damage.

Today, I believe that B12 supplementation is an important part of living a healthy vegan lifestyle. Let me prove to you why this is so by shattering the top eight myths surrounding this vitamin.

B12 Myth #1: Only vegans and vegetarians have to worry about B12 deficiency

Contrary to popular belief, vegans and vegetarians are not the only ones at risk for a B12 deficiency. The truth is, no matter what you eat, you could be at risk.

According to Sally Pacholok, R.N. and Jeffrey J. Stuart , D.O., authors of *Could It Be B12?*:

> ...while you need only a tiny, tiny amount of B12 each day (two to four micrograms or about a millionth of an ounce), it's remarkably easy to become deficient in this nutrient.
>
> While deficiency often occurs in vegans or vegetarians who fail to take the right supplements, *the majority of B12 deficient people eat plentiful amounts of the vitamin*-it's just that their bodies can't absorb or use it.[3]

The authors go on to say that the absorption process for B12 is very complex, more so than any other vitamin. Any disruption in this process will hinder B12 absorption.

And if the source of your B12 is meat, this adds an additional process because the B12 must be separated from the proteins in the meat that binds it. This is one possible explanation for why some meat-eaters ingesting plenty of B12 still struggle with getting enough of the vitamin.

Another step in the process involves intrinsic factor (IF), a glycoprotein that combines with B12 and carries the vitamin to the ileum for absorption. If you don't produce enough intrinsic factor—a condition known as pernicious anemia—you will not be able to absorb all of the B12 you consume.

Of course, there are other factors that affect intrinsic factor and your body's ability to absorb B12. Some of these unhealthy habits include drinking alcohol, smoking cigarettes, taking drugs (prescribed or otherwise), consuming an acid-forming diet of meat, dairy, and processed grains, eating frozen foods, and using colon cleansing products and procedures.

In summary, B12 deficiency tends to be the result of improper absorption, not inadequacy in the diet. This means that everyone, not just vegans and vegetarians, is at risk for deficiency.

And the science confirms this. In one study, researchers at Tufts University found that almost 40% of 3,000 individuals under the age of 50 had low B12 levels! And according to one of the researchers, "there were very few vegetarians in our study, and a lot were taking vitamin supplements."[4-5]

In another study, B12 status was analyzed in 340 Australian Seventh-day Adventist ministers. It's no surprise that the vegans and vegetarians in the group had low levels of B12, with approximately 73% below the lower limit of 221 pmol/L. But out of the 53 participants who consumed one or more servings of meat each week, 40% also had blood serum readings below this lower limit.[6]

B12 Myth #2: We can absorb plenty of B12 from bacteria in our intestines

Many vegan and raw vegans believe that bacteria in our intestines can be an adequate source of vitamin B12. As long as we avoid the unhealthy lifestyle practices that hinder absorption and destroy protective bacteria, we will have no need for supplementation.

As it turns out, many mammals do have the ability to absorb B12 synthesized by bacteria inhabiting their gut. According to the World Health Organization (WHO):

> **Most microorganisms, including bacteria and algae, synthesize vitamin B12, and they constitute the source of the vitamin...**

> In many animals, gastrointestinal fermentation supports the growth of these vitamin B12 synthesizing microorganisms, and subsequently the vitamin is absorbed and incorporated into the animal tissues.[7]

But what about human beings? Can we really absorb all the B12 we need from the bacteria in our gut?

It's very unlikely.

As I mentioned in the first myth, vitamin B12 is absorbed in the ileum, the last section of the small intestine. This is a problem because the majority of the bacteria that synthesize B12 live in the large intestine. It's very unlikely that we can absorb this B12 produced in our large intestine.[8]

Many vegans will counteract this point by referencing non-human wild primates like gorillas and bonobos. These creatures have the same basic anatomical structure that we do, consume a diet of fruit and vegetation, yet seem to have no issues with B12 deficiency.

The only explanation, claim these individuals, is that these primates are manufacturing the B12 themselves.

First, none of these animals consume a vegan or even a vegetarian diet. All of the great apes consume insects, and some of them even eat eggs and small invertebrates as well.[9]

Oh, and many primates—both in captivity and in the wild—have been observed eating their own feces, a practice called coprophagy. Disgusting as this may be to you or I, it is likely an excellent source of B12.

Second, these animals live in their natural environment. They are surrounded by trees, fresh air, pure water, and organic produce grown in fertile soils. They don't drink, smoke, take drugs, or participate in any other practices that may affect their ability to absorb the vitamin B12 they consume.

In other words, our primate cousins have plenty of opportunities to ingest B12—either from animal flesh, the soil itself, or their own and other animals' feces—AND their natural living practices ensure that they'll likely have no problems absorbing and utilizing it either.

On the other hand, we civilized humans do not have this luxury. We live in modern societies, surrounded by pollution, chemicals, stimulants, stressors, and "pristine" mass-produced produce grown in depleted soils.

And even if we do not smoke, drink, take drugs, or eat processed foods, most of us have spent the majority of our lives doing so.

Finally, the scientific evidence simply does not support the notion that healthy vegan humans can synthesize their own B12.

Take the following two-part study conducted in 1995, for instance. In the first part of the study, the researchers compared "serum vitamin B12 concentrations" (aka the amount of B12 in the blood) in 21 raw vegans with that of 21 omnivores.

Not only were the raw vegans' levels lower than that of the meat-eaters, but most of them had levels lower than the lower reference limit of 200 pmol/L (the mean was 193 pmol/L).[10]

The findings from the second part of the study were even more significant. In this longitudinal study, the researchers analyzed blood samples from nine raw vegans over a two-year period. During this time, B12 serum levels dropped in all but one of the participants!

Of the three subjects who still had B12 levels within the healthy range after the two years, two of them were eating exorbitant amounts of seaweed (either Nori or Chorella). I'll get to why this is not a recommended practice for B12 intake in a moment.

For now, suffice it to say that if you are consuming a raw vegan diet without some form of B12 supplementation, it is more than likely that you are or will become deficient in this vital nutrient. If you're relying upon intestinal bacteria to fulfill your needs, you might as well be wishing upon a star.

B12 Myth #3: Vegans require less B12

I know what you're thinking: so what if raw vegans have lower B12 levels? We also tend to have lower than normal white blood cell counts, blood pressure, protein, cholesterol, and urea levels, which are all signs of good health!

It makes perfect sense that vegans following a healthy, nutritionally adequate diet should have lower B12 levels without actually suffering from a B12 deficiency.

If this parallels your own thinking, you certainly aren't alone. Here's what Dr. Colin T. Campbell, renowned author of *The China Study*, has to say on this issue:

> Clearly, vegans do generally have lower blood concentrations of B12. A number of studies have shown this. But these low concentrations mean little unless there is a higher incidence of the accompanying blood (megaloblastic anemia) and nerve (parathesia) disorders, for which there seems to be little or no evidence.
>
> What should be acknowledged is that the concentrations of other blood factors, such as cholesterol, also are very different among vegans, and for very good health reasons at that. Why should we expect the lower B12 levels to be an exception?[11]

And here's one from Dr. John A. McDougall, creator of the low fat, starch-based McDougall Program:

> All these conditions caused by a B12-sufficient diet are found in the people you live and work with daily. How many vegans have you met with B12 deficiency anemia or nervous system damage? I bet not one! Furthermore, you have never even heard of such a problem unless you have read the attention-seeking headlines of newspapers or medical journals.[12]

While it may be true that you and I have never heard of met vegetarians/vegans suffering from these deadly disorders, how many of us have heard countless tales of vegans struggling with fatigue, mental fogginess, numbness/tingling in the hands and feet, and other symptoms of mild B12 deficiency?

Stories just like this one represented in "Vitamin B12: Are Your Getting It?":

> For the last few months, I was feeling sluggish, had to lie down a couple of times a day, found it difficult to work evenings and to exercise for long periods. Under [my vegan, medical doctor's] guidance, I was taking protein powder, creatine, testosterone, nystatin, etc., all to no avail. I was taking nutritional yeast every day, so I knew it wasn't B12 deficiency.

> Then, one day, I came across your B12 article by sheer accident. I wasn't going to read the whole thing, but I glanced through it and was struck by your insistence that none of the usual sources are adequate. I still didn't believe it, but I had some old B12 pills in the fridge, so I popped one.

> The effect was almost immediate and remarkable. I have been taking them almost every day, my stamina and energy level are up, and I feel middle-aged again instead of a tired old man.[13]

In summary, I think it's possible that healthy vegans require less B12. I just don't think this is likely for most of us. And regardless of Campbell and McDougall's musings, both ultimately recommend B12 supplementation for anyone following a diet devoid of animal products.

B12 Myth #4: Sea Veggies are a great source of B12

Remember the study on B12 status in raw vegans I mentioned earlier? You know, the one in which the vegans who consumed large amounts of seaweeds on a regular basis had blood B12 readings twice as high as those who didn't?

Here's what the researchers had to say about it:

> **The concentrations of vitamin B-12 in the serum of the subjects using large amounts of Chlorella (subject #9) or Nori (subject #6) were clearly above the mean of the vegan group.**
>
> **...However, this practice is not recommended, because excessive use of these seaweeds will concomitantly lead to harmful amounts of dietary iodine.**[10]

But an overdose of iodine isn't the only reason to limit seaweed consumption. As it turns out, eating seaweed to improve vitamin B12 levels can actually have the opposite effect!

That's because sea veggies contain various inactive B12 analogues that are not usable by the body and may actually interfere with the absorption of "true" B12.[12]

And a simple serum B12 test cannot distinguish between inactive and active B12 (more on that in a moment). So even though the two participants eating large amounts of seaweeds had higher serum B12 readings, we don't know how much of this B12 was actually being absorbed and assimilated into their tissues and cells.

But it gets worse.

In 1999, Japanese researchers wanted to see if Nori consumption could reduce methylmalonic acid levels (MMA) in humans. An increase in MMA is a sure sign of B12 deficiency, unlike a blood serum B12 test.

So these researchers conducted a urinary methylmalonic acid (uMMA) test on ten participants, gave them either dried or raw nori for three to nine days, then tested again.

The result?

Neither the raw nor the dried nori decreased uMMA levels in any of the patients. In both cases, levels actually increased! The raw nori raised uMMA by a mere 5% while the dried nori raised uMMA by a whopping 77%![13]

From the research we have now, seaweed—other than dulse, which hasn't been studied enough—simply isn't a reliable source of vitamin B12.

B12 Myth #5: We can get plenty of B12 from organic plants grown in B12-rich soils

In 1994, a study was conducted by Swedish researchers testing the ability of certain plants to uptake B12 from soils known to contain the vitamin. Not only were these plants—spinach, soybean, and barley—fully capable of absorbing B12, but the plants grown with organic fertilizers absorbed even more.[14]

This is great news! All we have to do is just eat more organically grown fruits and vegetables and we'll get plenty of B12!

Not necessarily.

The study only tells us that these plants are able to uptake B12 via the soil. What it does not tell us is what form the B12 is in. This B12 could be inactive, as it is in many seaweeds. In this case, it would not be useful to the body and could actually interfere with the absorption of usable B12, as I explained in the previous myth.

It would be wonderful if we could get all the B12 we need simply by eating more organically grown fruits and veggies, but there isn't any science to support this. No studies have been done showing whether or not consumption of these foods has the power to reduce uMMA levels and eradicate B12 deficiency in humans.

B12 Myth #6: There's plenty of B12 in human bodily fluids

Oh, you haven't heard this one? Boy, is it a doozy!

Basically, some vegans believe that human semen is rich in vitamin B12. So instead of supplementation, all we vegans need to do is…

Well, I'll let Robert Cohen from notmilk.com lay it out for you:

> **Vegan blood contains some B-12. In that, there is no debate. Vegan semen and vaginal secretions contain many times more Vitamin B-12 than does human blood.**
>
> **The solution? Make love. Enjoy oral sex. The ingestion of sexual body secretions from your significant other will insure good health for you through a Biblically-endorsed version of vegan nutrition.**[15]

Semen and vaginal secretions rich in B12, huh? I did a bit of digging and as it turns out, what tends to be present in large amounts in male semen is transcobalamin II.

What is transcobalamin II? It's a carrier protein that binds to cobalamin. Contrary to Cohen's statement above, cobalamin (aka vitamin B12) is found in roughly the same amount that is present in human blood.[16]

As far as vaginal fluid also being rich in vitamin B12, I could not find one piece of literature confirming this statement. I'll just chalk that one up to more wishful thinking.

B12 Myth #7: My blood test was normal so I don't need to supplement

If you go to a physician to get your B12 levels checked, you will most likely receive a serum B12 test. This is a simple blood test that checks for the amount of B12 present in your blood.

The problem here is that a serum B12 test only tells you how much B12 is in your blood, not whether this B12 is active or inactive or how much B12 is actually being used by the body.

And as we already learned, B12 deficiency is typically caused by malabsorption, not inadequate B12 in the diet. Luckily, there is a better test. It's called the urinary Methylmalonic Acid Test (uMMA).

By using this test, studies have shown that it is possible to have serum B12 levels within the normal range (200-400 pmol/L) and yet still have elevated uMMA levels.[17-18] In other words, the serum B12 test cleared these individuals for a B12 deficiency, while the more accurate uMMA test proved that they were indeed deficient!

So why is a uMMA test a better judge of a B12 deficiency? As I mentioned above, all the serum B12 test can do is tell you how much B12 is in your blood. The uMMA test, however, tells you how much methylmalonic acid is in your urine.

This is important because the amount of MMA in your body is dependent upon B12.

In a normal human body with adequate B12, the B12 acts as a co-factor in the conversion of methylmalonic acid to succinyl-CoA. But if you aren't absorbing enough B12, some of the MMA will not be converted and so your levels of MMA will be higher than normal.[19]

So just because your serum B12 levels are within the normal range does not mean that you are not deficient in B12. If you want to be certain, get yourself a uMMA test.

B12 Myth #8: A supplement can never be as good as nutrition from whole foods

This is true. But as I've tried to show you with this article, the likelihood that we can get enough B12 from our foods is slim to none.

And while one vitamin that has been isolated and packed into a pill is inferior to that same vitamin found in fresh foods, along with all the other nutrients that would accompany it, that doesn't mean that B12 supplements don't work. We know that a quality sublingual or oral B12 supplement will raise most people's MMA levels.

The other issue people have with supplements is that they are afraid of taking too much.

This is really a moot point when it comes to B12, perhaps more than any other nutritional supplement. No toxic side effects have been associated with oral supplementations or intramuscular injections, even at megadoses of 9,000 mcg per day! *[20]

Plus, it's been shown that at doses of 200-2,000 mcg per day taken orally, only about 1% of the B12 is absorbed.[20] The average daily oral supplement contains 1,000 mcg, so at an absorption rate of 1%, only 10 mcg would actually be used by the body.

Take Action

Ditch the dogma and get yourself a uMMA test. If your levels are high (above 3.8 micrograms of MMA per milligram of creatinine), begin supplementation and test again in two months to see if your levels have been reduced.

If your MMA levels are fine, you don't have to worry about supplementation. However, it is imperative that you continue to get tested on a regular basis, preferably once per year, but at least every three years. Just because you are not deficient now does not mean that you won't be in the future.

If you have not had any B12 source for a while, Registered Dietician and author of *Vegan For Life* Jack Norris recommends taking 2,000 mcg of cyanocobalamin once a day for two weeks. For maintenance,

* While taking large doses of 1,000 mcg per day for several months, I started to breakout a little bit on my face and upper back. The breakouts stopped a couple months after stopping supplementation and have not returned since I started taking the dosage recommended on the following page. There are a few other cases of acne and rosacea occurring with large supplemental doses of B12 as well.[21-23]

take two doses of 2-3.5 mcg per day, one dose of 25-100 mcg per day, or two doses of 1,000 mcg per week.[24]

There are plenty of adequate B12 supplements on the market today so I won't list any specific brands here. Both cyanocobalamin and methylcobalamin appear to effective at raising at raising MMA levels, but methylcobalamin may require larger doses.[25]

Again, the important thing is to get retested to make sure the supplement and dosage are working to lower your methylmalonic acid levels. If your MMA levels have not lowered to some degree after two months of supplementation, try another brand or up your dosage.

This Ain't Your Mama's Produce

Supplement companies will tell you that today's fruits and vegetables are much lower in nutrients than they should be. Modern-day agricultural practices have left are soils severely depleted and if the nutrients aren't in the soil, they won't be in the plant.

While these companies tend to exaggerate in an effort to scare you into buying their pills and powders, there's no doubt that today's produce is less nutritious than it once was.

In one study published in 2004, researchers from the University of Texas examined nutritional data from 1950 and 1999 for 43 different fruits and vegetables.[26] They found that on the whole, amounts of vitamin c, riboflavin, protein, calcium, phosphorus, and iron had all declined. The team also suspected declines in other nutrients including magnesium and zinc, but could not confirm because these minerals were not reported in 1950.

The reason for the decline?

> **We suggest that any real declines are generally most easily explained by changes in cultivated varieties between 1950 and 1999, in which there may be trade-offs between yield and nutrient content."[26]**

Another study found similar results. Of twenty fruits and twenty-one vegetables, "there were significant reductions in the levels of Ca [calcium], Mg [magnesium], Cu [copper], and Na [sodium], in vegetables and Mg [magnesium], Fe [iron], Cu [copper], and K [potassium] in fruits."[27]

The reason for the decline?

> Agriculture which relies on NPK [Nitrogen-Phosphorus-Potassium] fertilizers and pesticides, that adds little organic matter to the soil and that alternates between soil compaction and ploughing, could produce food depleted in minerals. These practices affect the structure, chemistry and ecology of the soil in ways that could affect the availability of minerals to plants and hence the mineral content of crops.[27]

What About Organic?

Contrary to popular belief, organic fruits and vegetables are not necessarily more nutritious than their conventionally grown counterparts.

In fact, according to one review that examined 162 articles published between 1958 and 2008, "no evidence of a difference in nutrient quality between organically and conventionally produced foodstuffs" for most nutrients.[28]

A more recent review found that while organic foods are 30% less likely to be contaminated with pesticides, there is little evidence that they are significantly more nutritious than conventionally grown produce.[29]

What's going on here?

In the United States, the "USDA Certified Organic" label means:

1) No sewage sludge[30]
2) No genetic modification[30]
3) No antibiotics[30]
4) No prohibited substances*[30]
5) No irradiation[30]

This doesn't tell you anything about the nutrients in the soil or whether or not the food was picked too early. If the soil is depleted, the food will be too. If the food is picked too early, it will not have gotten a chance to absorb all of the nutrients it would have if it had remained on the vine, on the tree, or in the ground longer.

Relying on organic produce to get all the nutrients you need simply isn't enough.

The Solution?

Multivitamin/mineral (MVM) supplements.

A quality supplement containing moderate amounts of essential vitamins and minerals (e.g. thiamin, riboflavin, folate, zinc, iron, selenium, etc.) will help make up for small amounts that may be lacking in a healthy raw food diet.

If you don't mind taking a supplement that contains animal products like gelatin and lanolin-derived D3, the options are almost endless. Looking for supplements that have been independently tested and approved by private companies and organizations like ConsumerLab. com, the National Sanitation Foundation (NSF), and the United States Pharmacopeia (USP) is a good place to start.

If you want to take a supplement devoid of all animal products and derivatives, then your options are much more limited. Luckily, a few vegan MVM supplements are available such as VeganLife, DEVA Nutrition, VegLife, and Pure Vegan.

---

* Prohibited substances include most synthetic substances and some natural ones like arsenic and tobacco dust.

Since you should meet the vast majority of your nutritional needs just by eating a fresh fruit and vegetable diet, I recommend taking your MVM every 2-3 days instead of daily.

What About Nutrient Toxicity?

Opponents of supplementation almost always point to toxicity as the main reason to avoid supplements. They argue that taking any nutrient in supplement form puts you at risk of overdosing.

What these individuals often neglect to point out is that signs of nutrient toxicity almost always involve very high doses, doses much higher than what is found in your average MVM supplement.

Here are some examples.

Iron

Iron at 50 mg per day can cause gastrointestinal distress like nausea, vomiting, and diarrhea.[31] Your average MVM supplement contains 18 mg or less per serving.

Copper

Copper at 4 mg per day can cause gastrointestinal distress.[31] Your average MVM supplement contains 2 mg or less per serving.

Beta-Carotene

Beta-carotene at 20 mg per day (33,333 IU) and greater has been associated with increased risk for lung cancer.[32] Your average MVM supplement contains 5,000 IU or less per serving.*

Selenium

Selenium above 850 mcg/day can cause hair and nail loss, skin rashes, and gastrointestinal distress.[32] Your average MVM supplement contains 200 mcg or less per serving.

---

* Most MVM supplements contain 5,000 IU or more of vitamin A either from preformed vitamin A, plant-based carotenoids like beta-carotene, or a combination of the two. If your MVM is vegan, it will not contain any preformed vitamin A (retinol) which is sourced from animal products only. It will likely contain betacarotene only or a combination of various carotenoids.

In other words, a quality MVM supplement is safe. And remember, I recommend taking only 1/4-1/2 of the recommend dosage.*

Vitamin D: Is Sunshine Really Enough?

Vitamin D is perhaps the most talked about nutrient right now, and with good reason. Not only is it needed for strong bones, vitamin D deficiency has also been linked to virtually every major health concern, including heart disease, hypertension, obesity, rheumatoid arthritis, dementia, and several types of cancer.[34, 35, 36, 37, 38, 39-40]

But unlike with true essential vitamins, food and supplements are not the only sources of vitamin D. That's because your body actually synthesizes vitamin D—which is actually a hormone precursor called a secosteroid—from exposure to sunlight.

But what about those of us on a vitamin D-free raw vegan diet? Will soaking up some sun be enough to produce adequate amounts of vitamin D?

Before I can answer these questions, let's see how much vitamin D we really need in the first place.

Ideal Vitamin D Levels

There are two main sides to the vitamin D debate.

1) Those who believe that vitamin D is necessary for bone health and bone health alone

2) Those who believe that vitamin D is an incredibly powerful nutrient that can protect us from all kinds of diseases and disorders beyond bone health

---

* Some MVM supplements do contain potentially harmful amounts of certain B vitamins. For example, Deva's vegan multivitamin contains 50 mg of niacin and yet the tolerable upper intake level (UL) is 35 mg per day.[33] This isn't a concern if you take one serving every 2-3 days instead of daily.

Bone Health

The Institute of Medicine holds that a serum vitamin D level of 20 nanograms per milliliter is sufficient for skeletal health.[41] However, there is quite a bit of evidence suggesting that this is too low and that the threshold should really be closer to 30 ng/mL.[42-45]

Because of all of this research, experts like Dr. Michael F. Holick, author of *The Vitamin D Solution*, and the International Osteoporosis Foundation recommend a threshold of 30 ng/mL for bone health.[46-48]

Non-Skeletal Benefits

Numerous epidemiological studies have found that having a vitamin D level closer to 40 ng/mL offers decreased risks for breast, prostate, and colorectal cancer, poor dental health, diabetes, and multiple sclerosis.[42, 48, 49, 50, 51]

However, not all studies have shown these connections. For instance, one study found that even at high levels of 70 ng/mL, vitamin D did not prevent diabetes in those at high risk for becoming diabetic.[52]

There is even some evidence that higher vitamin D levels could be harmful. In one recent observational study that analyzed vitamin D levels from almost 250,000 Copenhageners, subjects with a vitamin D level of 56 ng/mL or greater had a 42% greater risk of dying during the study than did subjects with a level of 20 ng/mL.[53]

Confused? Me too. But there is one more factor I think we should take into account before settling on an optimal vitamin D level.

The Sun-Worshipping Ways of Our Ancestors

Like our primate cousins, humans have evolved to thrive in tropical climates. Our hunter-gatherer ancestors spent everyday outdoors, soaking up tons of sunlight year-round. As a result, they likely had vitamin D levels that were significantly higher than today's average American.[54]

There is even evidence that supports this hypothesis. A study published in January 2012 found that for 35 Maasai and 25 Hadzabe, pastoralists and hunter-gatherers living in East Africa, mean vitamin D levels were 48 (range 23-67) and 44 (range 28-68) ng/mL, respectively.[55]

So What is Optimal?

Frankly, I don't know.

What I do know is that less than 20 ng/mL is very likely too low for skeletal health. There is evidence to show and many experts agree that less than 30 ng/mL is still too low. From my own personal experience, I'm confident that less than 30 ng/mL is too low to ensure proper calcium absorption and skeletal health in my own body.

Finally, less than 40 ng/mL may still be too low based on our own tropical heritage and for disease prevention. With all of this in mind, I personally shoot for a vitamin D level of 40-60 ng/mL.*

Now that we have a better idea of where our vitamin D levels should be for optimal health, let's find out how much sun exposure we need to meet this levels.

Ideal Sun Exposure

Unfortunately, there's no one-size-fits-all recommendation for everyone regarding sun exposure. There are just too many factors that affect vitamin D availability and absorption, such as skin type, location, age, and, body weight.

Fortunately, figuring out your own exposure needs is pretty easy.

In his book *The Vitamin D Solution*, Dr. Holick recommends sunning your arms and legs for 25-50% of the time it takes for your skin to

---

* This range is mostly based on the likelihood that our ancestors had levels of 40 ng/mL or more. I'm personally not too concerned about the other possible benefits of higher vitamin D levels like diabetes and colon cancer. My healthy eating and exercise habits alone significantly reduce my chances of getting these and other modern day diseases.

turn slightly pink. You should do this two to three days per week between the hours of 11am and 3pm.[46]

If you have type 1 skin (very fair, always burns), this will take roughly 1-5 minutes in a subtropical climate (25-35 degrees latitude) during the summer months.[*] If you have type 3 skin (occasionally burns and gradually tans), it will take 10-15 minutes.[**][46]

No sunscreen should be worn during this time since it significantly reduces vitamin D production.55-56 However, Dr. Holick does recommend using sunscreen (ideally SPF30) for any additional sun exposure you receive to reduce the risk of non-melanoma skin cancer and wrinkles.[46]

Does the Sun Really Cause Skin Cancer?

While some may argue that small doses of intentional sun exposure are safe, dermatologists point out that the risk of developing skin cancer from ultraviolet (UV) radiation far outweighs the benefit of stimulating vitamin D production – particularly when enriched foods and supplements are safe and effective sources of this vitamin. ~American Academy of Dermatology

The connection between sun exposure and skin cancer is not as cut-and-dried as the American Academy of Dermatology would have us believe. Yes, excess sun exposure will cause skin damage and even skin cancer. However, this is non-melanoma skin cancer we're talking about, which is both easy to detect and to treat.[58-59]

Melanoma, the most deadly form of skin cancer, has *no direct connection to sun exposure.* In fact, regular sun exposure likely helps protect against the development of melanoma!60-61 Studies have found that people who work outdoors have a lower risk for developing the disease.[60 & 62]

Plus, there is evidence that antioxidants like selenium and beta-carotene protect against sunburn.[63-64] Since adopting an antioxidant-rich raw food diet, I have noticed that I do not burn as easily as I once did.

---

[*]   Check out *www.knowyourskintype.com* for more info on determining your skin type.

[**]   Check out *www.whatsmylatling.com* to find out your area's latitude.

Finally, one study found that subjects with a history of non-melanoma skin cancer who ate a low-fat diet (less than 21%) for two years experienced significantly less pre-cancerous skin growths than those who ate 36% or more of their calories from fat.[65] A low fat raw vegan diet is, of course, low in fat!

In conclusion, there's no doubt that excessive exposure to sunlight causes skin damage and even cancer. However, there's no evidence that the amounts of sun exposure necessary to optimize vitamin D levels cause skin cancer.[58]

So Sunshine is Enough?

There's no doubt that it is possible to get enough vitamin D from sun exposure alone. However, there are a few factors that may keep your body from producing enough of this essential vitamin/hormone.

Skin Color

The darker your skin tone, the more melanin your body produces. The more melanin your body produces, the more protection you will have against sun damage, but the less vitamin D you will be able to synthesize from sunlight exposure.

According to Dr. Holick, someone with type 5 or 6 skin (dark skin, rarely or never burns) will need 20-30 minutes of sun exposure three times per week in a subtropical climate during the summer months.[46] That's 3-4 times the amount required by someone with type 2 skin (fair, burns easily), but it's still only 60-90 minutes a week.

UV Index

Just because you are spending lots of time in the sunshine doesn't mean you are producing enough (or any) vitamin D. That's because vitamin D production actually requires exposure to UVB rays, and these are only present in sufficient quantities when the UV index is greater than three.

Unless you live in the tropics, it's very likely that there will be times during the year when the UV index is three or less. In the United States, most states have a low UV index from November to February.[*][66]

So for many of us, it's very important to get adequate sun exposure (see guidelines above) during the summer months when the UV index is high enough.

Age

It's well-known that aging reduces the body's ability to produce vitamin D.[68]

Weight

There is some evidence that being overweight decreases bioavailability of vitamin D.[68-69] A study published in September 2000 found that subjects with a body mass index (BMI) of 30 or greater had an increase in vitamin D3 that was 57% lower than the subjects with a BMI of 25 or less.[69]

Of course, as I pointed out in chapter three, you shouldn't have any concerns about becoming or staying obese on a healthy fruit- and vegetable-based raw food diet.

So Sunshine Isn't Enough?

Sunshine is definitely enough if you get enough. But how can you know for sure if you're getting enough?

The best way to find out if you're producing enough vitamin D is to get tested. The test you want is the 25-hydroxy-vitamin D (25 OH vitamin D) test. It's a simple blood test that your doctor can do for you or that you can do yourself at home.

---

[*]   Here's a tip from the Vitamin D Council. If your shadow is longer than you are tall, your body is not producing much vitamin D.[67]

At the very least, shooting for at least 30 ng/mL (75 nmol/L) for bone health is a good idea. As I already said, I personally aim for 40-60 ng/mL (100-150 nmol/L).

An indirect way of testing for vitamin D is to check your calcium levels. In 2011, I got some blood work done and both my vitamin D and calcium were low (24 ng/mL and 8.3 mg/dL). I began supplementation with vitamin D *without taking a calcium supplement or making any changes to my diet.* Three months later, both my vitamin D and calcium had risen to normal levels (48 ng/mL and 9 mg/dL).

Why would vitamin D effect calcium levels?

Because vitamin D is required for proper calcium absorption.69 In fact, one study found that when postmenopausal women with a mean vitamin D level of 20 ng/mL increased their level to 35 ng/mL, calcium absorption increased by 45-65%![71]

So if your calcium levels are low yet your calcium intake is adequate, it may be because vitamin D is low. Increase your vitamin D levels via sunlight or supplements (see guidelines below) and get retested in 2-3 months. If your vitamin D and calcium levels rise, this is a good sign that you were not getting enough vitamin D.

Should We Supplement?

According to Dr. Holick, if you get plenty of sun during the summer, even if you live at a high latitude (50-75 degrees), it's possible to produce enough vitamin D without supplementation. However, supplementation is a great backup plan to make sure your vitamin D levels remain high enough even during the colder months.[46]

Dr. Holick recommends 1,000-2,000 IU per day to ensure vitamin D levels of at least 30 ng/mL.[46] While I live at a subtropical latitude (35 degrees) and have access to D-producing sunshine for most months during the year, I personally take a vitamin D supplement from November to February.

D3 or D2?

There are two forms of vitamin D: cholecalciferol (D3) and ergocalciferol (D2). D3 is produced from lanolin, a substance found in sheep's wool, and D2 is produced from fungi.[*]

While several studies have shown D3 to be more effective at raising vitamin D levels, others have shown them to be equally effective.[72-74, 75-77] As vegan and Registered Dietician Jack Norris points out, many of the studies showing D3 to be more effective involved large, infrequent doses (e.g. one dose of 50,000 IU) while the studies showing equal effectiveness used smaller, more frequent doses (e.g. 1,000 IU/day).[77]

Most experts agree that taking a D2 supplement will raise your vitamin D levels.[**78-79] You just may have to take more of it than you would D3, perhaps as much as 2.5 times more.[80]

When to Take Vitamin D?

Vitamin D is a fat-soluble vitamin so it makes since that consuming it with fat will improve absorption. While one study did find a positive correlation between vitamin D absorption and monounsaturated fats, the improvement was small.[81]

However, when you take your vitamin D supplement may still matter.

One study examined 17 men and women who, despite taking supplements, were vitamin D deficient. Some were taking average-sized doses (1,000 IU/day), others were taking megadoses (50,000 IU/day), but all were taking their supplements on an empty stomach or with a small meal.[82]

The researchers instructed the subjects to keep taking their usual supplement and dose, but to start taking it with their largest meal of the day. After 2-3 months, the average vitamin D level increased by over 50% (from 30.5 to 47.2 ng/mL)![82]

---

[*]   A vegan D3 supplement produced from lichens is now on the market. It's called Vitashine and is available in spray and capsule form.

[**]   Please don't just assume that your vitamin D supplement is working for you. If you're deficient, keep getting tested until you reach healthy levels and continue to get tested on a regular basis (i.e. yearly).

Granted this is only one study, a rather small one, and one that didn't use a control group. But if you've been struggling to reach optimal vitamin D levels despite adequate vitamin D intake, taking your supplement with your largest meal of the day may help.

Toxicity?

Too much vitamin D from supplements (it's impossible to overdose from sun exposure) can cause a condition called hypercalcemia, or too much calcium in the blood, which can then cause nausea, vomiting, kidney stones, kidney failure, and osteoporosis.[83-84]

To prevent hypercalcemia, the Institute of Medicine (IOM) has set a tolerable upper intake level (UL) for vitamin D at 4,000 IU per day.[41] Following Dr. Holick's recommendation of 1,000-2,000 IU per day will keep you well below the toxic threshold.

That said, this threshold is likely too low. The vast majority of vitamin D intoxication cases have involved doses of 50,000 IU or more.[40] There's no evidence that I am aware of that taking doses of 5,000 or even 10,000 IU a day will result in vitamin D toxicity.

A much more accurate UL for vitamin D is likely 10,000 IU or more. Even the IOM admits that "doses below 10,000 IU/day are not usually associated with toxicity" and "most reports suggest that the toxicity threshold is between 10,000 and 40,000 IU of vitamin D per day."[41]

In terms of vitamin D levels, toxicity typically manifests at 200-240 ng/mL or higher.[41] This is at least four times the levels that the average person getting plenty of summer sun and taking 1,000-2,000 IU/day during the colder months will experience.[41]

Why Not Just Supplement?

When you are exposed to sunlight, you make not only vitamin D but also at least five and up to ten additional photoproducts that you would never get from dietary sources or from a supplement. So the obvious question is, why would Mother Nature be making all of these vitamin D photoproducts if they weren't having a biological effect? ~ Dr. Micheal F. Holick, The Vitamin D Solution

Most of us know that when it comes to meeting our nutrient needs from pills versus getting them from fruits and vegetables, there's no comparison. Supplements simply can't provide all of the water, fiber, and thousands of phytonutrients that are found in one apple, head of romaine lettuce, or bunch of grapes.

It's the same with vitamin D and sunshine. Exposing your skin to the sun's rays provides more than just vitamin D, including the fact that it just feels good! A vitamin D supplement provides vitamin D and only vitamin D.

However, for those with type 1 skin who always burn easily no matter how much sun they get, relying on supplementation exclusively may be helpful. But remember that you can still get some sun even if you have type 1 skin. At subtropical latitudes, you'll likely only need 1-5 minutes during the summer months from 11am-3pm to produce enough vitamin D for the year.[46]

Sunshine + Supplements = Skeletal Health and Beyond

Michael Pollan, author of *In Defense of Food: An Eater's Manifesto*, has a very popular saying that goes like this:

Eat food. Not too much. Mostly plants.

With regards to vitamin D, I think we could revise this to say:

Get sun. Not too much. Don't forget to supplement.

Expose your arms and legs for 25-50% of the time it takes for your skin to turn slightly pink two to three days per week between the hours of 11am and 3pm. Take 1,000-2,000 IU/day of vitamin D (D2 or D3) during the colder months.

Following Dr. Holick's guidelines, you should have no trouble maintaining a vitamin D level of at least 30 ng/mL.

Better Safe Than Sorry

No, supplements are not ideal. The ideal scenario would be to get all the nutrients you need from the food you eat. This may not be a reality for most of us, but that isn't to say that it's impossible.

If you have access to a variety of fruits and vegetables grown in nutrient-rich soils and live an otherwise healthy lifestyle that includes adequate sunshine, sleep, fresh water, and clean air (among other health factors), while also avoiding stress and pollutants, then it may be possible that you don't need supplementation.

For the rest of us, I believe supplementation to be an important part of thriving on a healthy raw vegan diet.*

Fruits and Veggies Are Still Fantastic Foods

I don't want to give you the impression that fruits and vegetables are not healthy foods. Quite the contrary!

The following is a quote from that 50-year review on organics I mentioned earlier:

> **Plant cells require most human nutrients for their own functioning. They cannot grow, much less be viable commercial food crops, without synthesizing or acquiring their own needed levels of a broad range of nutrients... Currently available vegetables and fruits are still our most broadly nutrient-dense foods, and hundreds of studies document their superior health-promoting qualities.**[26]

In other words, today's fruits and vegetables are still the healthiest foods available. They're high in various vitamins and minerals, full of phytochemicals, and low in fat and toxins.

---

* Please don't just assume that this describes your lifestyle. Get regular blood work done to confirm.

Food First, Supplements Second

Supplements, no matter how well-made, cannot replace a poor diet. If you eat a diet high in calories and low in nutrients, supplements aren't going to help you much. A pill can't undo the damage of nutritional excess.

Also, supplements created in a lab can only contain *known* nutrients. This would be great if we knew all of the nutrients present in our foods, but we don't.

Eating a diet predominated by fresh fruits and vegetables and supplementing with a multivitamin/mineral, B12, and D supplement offers the best of both worlds.

CHAPTER 8
Health Isn't Just About What You Eat

In some of the preceding chapters, you may have noticed that I sometimes use the phrase "raw food lifestyle" in place "raw food diet".

Why? Because health isn't just about food.

Bummer, I know. If you truly want to experience optimal health and avoid degenerative disease, you have to give adequate attention to several other health factors, including...

Sleep

Approximately 30% of American workers (41 million) do not get enough sleep. This is particularly disturbing considering that lack of sleep is to blame for roughly 20% of car crashes and has been linked to weight gain, insulin resistance, and heart disease.[1, 2-4, 5-6, 7]

How Much Sleep is Enough?

Most experts agree that the average adult needs 7-9 hours of sleep per night.[8-9] If you feel refreshed and ready to go in the morning, you've likely had enough sleep. If you feel groggy or long for a nap during the day, you probably need more.

Tips for Sound Sleeping

Schedule Your Sleep

Choose a bedtime and stick with it, even on the weekends. This will help your body get on a schedule and will make getting to sleep, as well as waking up, easier.

Dark and Quiet

Your bedroom should be as dark and as quiet as possible. Use an eye mask and ear plugs if necessary.

Comfort is Key

Invest in a good mattress and pillow. It doesn't have to be a Sleep Number or Tempur-Pedic, but it should be comfortable to you.

Work-Free Zone

Use your bed for sleeping only. No working in bed!

Turn Off the Toys

Avoid using your laptop, phone, tablet, or any device with a back-lit screen right before you go to sleep, as the light can suppress melatonin and disturb your sleep cycle. If you must play Angry Birds in bed, use the dimmest setting you can.

Avoid the Alarm

Waking up naturally without an alarm clock is the best way to go. If you must use an alarm, consider switching to a sun alarm clock. The "alarm" is a light that gradually gets brighter and brighter to simulate a natural sunrise.

I own the BioBrite Sunrise Clock and I love it. It's really great as a mellow reading light too.

Exercise

There's no doubt that we can't be truly healthy without physical activity. A proper exercise routine is so important for cardiovascular, bone, immune, and muscular health. It's also great for improving sleep, increasing energy, and boosting mood.

Not only that, there's also an abundance of evidence that exercise protects against diseases and disorders like type II diabetes, metabolic syndrome, colon cancer, breast cancer, and Parkinson's disease.[10, 11, 12, 13, 14]

While there is seemingly an infinite number of ways to stay active, there are two forms of exercise that I believe should form the basis for a well-rounded exercise routine.

#1: Strength Training

Strength training (aka resistance training) is absolutely vital for building and maintaining lean muscle mass and strong bones. It has also been shown to improve balance and insulin sensitivity, and reduce symptoms of depression.[15, 16, 17]

What Equipment Should I Use?

While weight lifting using dumbbells, barbells, or machines is the most common way to strength train, it's not the only way. You can use resistance bands, weighted balls (aka medicine balls), kettlebells, weighted vests, or even your own bodyweight!

What equipment you use isn't really important. What is important is that you use a resistance that's challenging. Typically, this means shooting for 2-3 sets of 8-12 repetitions per muscle group done 2-3 times per week.[*][**][***] Those last few repetitions should be a struggle to complete.

So if you can do 20 bicep curls using eight-pound dumbbells, increase the weight. Or if you can do 50 push ups on your toes, make the move harder by elevating your feet or staggering your hands.

Where Do I Start?

With all the free workouts and routines available on the internet,

---

[*] While one set may be adequate, there's evidence that 2-3 sets is optimal for strength gains.18-20 One study found that training for 2-3 sets per exercise resulted in 46% greater strength gains than training just one set per exercise![18]

[**] It's generally accepted that 8-12 repetitions per set is the best range for developing a balance of strength, hypertrophy (muscle size), and endurance, and for retaining or increasing bone mineral density.[21-22]

[***] It's also very important to rest at least 48 hours between muscle groups. So if you worked your chest and back on Monday, you wouldn't work them again until Wednesday or later.

getting started is pretty easy. A google search for "strength training for beginners" led me to a simple full body workout using only dumbbells and a stability ball from About.com (***www.exercise.about.com/cs/exbeginners/l/blbegstrength.htm***).

If you're a fitness dvd fanatic like I am, beginner strength training workouts are available. Collage Video (***www.collagevideo.com***) is an excellent resource, with clips and reviews of hundreds of workout dvds. I rarely ever purchase an exercise dvd without checking CV first.

#2: High-Intensity Interval Training

High-intensity interval training (HIIT), involves a brief period of maximal exertion (typically 20-60 seconds) followed by a brief period of active rest (typically 10-90 seconds) repeated for 4-20 minutes.

Here's an example.
- **Sprint as fast as you can for 30 seconds**
- **Jog or walk for 30 seconds**
- **Repeat 12 times**

That's just 12 minutes of work. 12 minutes of very intense, very difficult work, but still just 12 minutes total.

But time isn't the only thing that makes HIIT workouts so great. While steady-state aerobics like jogging and cycling are generally considered the best workouts for endurance, heart health, and burning body fat, interval training offers all that and more.[23, 24]

HIIT Improves Endurance

There is ample evidence that interval workouts are excellent for endurance training.[24 & 25-28] In fact, one study found that recreationally active individuals who participated in sprint interval training over two weeks (a total of just 15 minutes of actual work) were able to increase their cycle endurance capacity by 100%![29]

HIIT Benefits the Heart

Research shows that short but intense interval workouts provide the same cardiovascular benefits as long but less-intense cardio workouts.[30] In fact, one study found that while both interval and "continuous" training reduced blood pressure, only interval training reduced arterial stiffness in patients with hypertension.[23]

High-intensity interval training is even recommended by some doctors for people with cardiovascular disease.[31]

HIIT Improves Insulin Sensitivity

High-intensity interval training is incredibly effective at improving insulin sensitivity.[28] & [32-35] A study published in 2011 found that when seven sedentary individuals completed just six sessions of HIIT in two weeks, insulin sensitivity improved by about 35% after training.[33]

HIIT Burns More Fat

There's no doubt that HIIT workouts are fabulous for fat loss.[32 & 36-39] In one study of eight women, just seven sessions of HIIT over 13 days increased fat oxidation by 36%![36]

One of the things that makes HIIT so effective for fat loss is its ability to burn so many calories, even more than a typical aerobic workout.

But how in the world can working out for 30 minutes or less burn more calories than working out for 60? It has to do with something called excess-post exercise oxygen consumption (EPOC), or the "after-burn" effect.

Even though you burn significantly less calories during a short HIIT workout than you do during a long aerobic workout, the anaerobic (without oxygen) nature of HIIT creates an oxygen debt that your body then has to work to repay. This extra work means your body is burning more calories for several hours after your workout (after-burn), perhaps as much as 48 hours later!*[40-41]

---

*   Remember, you can workout all you want but if your diet is poor, you likely won't reach your ideal weight. A healthy low fat, high carb, raw food diet coupled with a balanced work-out routine makes reaching and maintaining your ideal weight almost effortless.

No wonder high-intensity interval training is all the rage these days!

Getting Started

Although traditionally used by athletes, anyone can use HIIT to maximize performance and get in shape.* You just have to start slowly and listen to your body.

Here's a simple routine for beginners:

- **Run as fast as you can for 10-15 seconds****
- **Walk for 90-120 seconds**
- **Repeat one more time or stop**

Make sure you warm up with some light cardio for 3-5 minutes beforehand. Keep progressing each time you do the workout by increasing the time you run, decreasing the time you rest, or adding more rounds.

The key here, and with any HIIT routine, is that you're working as hard as YOU can. This may mean a full sprint or it may mean a light jog. It doesn't matter as long as you're working at your maximum.

Too Much is Unhealthy, Too!

Exercise has its rewards, but it also has its risks. Vigorous exercise puts a lot of stress on the body, especially the knees and ankles, and causes oxidative stress.

For active individuals working out for 30-60 minutes per day, the pros of exercising far outweigh any cons.

For the very active, particularly endurance athletes, this may not be the case. Excessive exercise increases the risk for overuse injuries and has been linked to heart damage, abnormal heart rhythms, low bone mineral density, and amenorrhea (no menstruation) in women.[42-43, 44-46, 47]

---

*   If you're new to exercise of any kind, it's probably best to start with low to moderate-intensity cardio exercise first. Once you can handle working at 60-85% of your maximum heart rate for 30 minutes or more, you're likely ready for HIIT.

**   High intensity doesn't have to mean high impact. There are plenty of ways you can have an effective interval workout without all the wear and tear on your joints. For instance, instead of sprinting on concrete, sprint on a rebounder or in a pool.

Stress Management

Essentially, we humans live well enough and long enough, and are smart enough, to generate all sorts of stressful events purely in our heads. How many hippos worry about whether Social Security is going to last as long as they will, or what they are going to say on a first date? ~ Robert M. Sapolsky, Why Zebra Don't Get Ulcers

For most animals, stress is a short-term response to a simple stressor. In the case of the lion chasing the gazelle, both animals experience stress. Once the chase is over, whether the lion catches the zebra or the zebra escapes, the stress dissipates for both animals.

While we humans don't have to worry about eating or being eaten, we do worry about bills, relationships, and whether or not our team will make the playoffs this year.

The problem with this modern-day stress is that it's long-lasting. If you're gritting your teeth over a presentation you have to give one month from now, that's one full month of stress. One full month versus the minutes, or even seconds that the human body has evolved to handle.

In *Why Zebras Don't Get Ulcers*, author Robert M. Sapolsky illustrates just how harmful this chronic psychological stress can be.[48] By undergoing long-term stress, you increase your risk for cardiovascular disease, type II diabetes, obesity, stomach ulcers, erectile dysfunction, amenorrhea, immune system suppression, and depression. Chronic stress may also be linked to type I diabetes, gastrointestinal disorders, osteoporosis, and even cancer.[48]

Where to Start?

Being super stressed was my Achilles' heal for a long time and from conquering it, I can tell you that learning how to decrease and manage stress is far beyond the scope of this book. Reading Sapolsky's book is a good start.

Is Stress Always Bad for Us?

Nope, not always.

Take exercise as an example. Lifting weights or sprinting up a hill is certainly stressful, but it's this stress that improves cardiovascular fitness, insulin sensitivity, and bone mineral density. It's good stress!

And physical activity is only one type of good stress, also known as eustress. Anticipating an upcoming event, being challenged at work, or solving a puzzle are all examples of good stress. They enliven our lives, keeping us challenged and fulfilled.

Without some stress, life would be pretty dull and boring.

Sleep, Exercise, Stress Management and...

Of course, there are other health factors besides diet, sleep, exercise, and stress management. Fresh air, clean water, adequate sunshine (which I covered in the last chapter), and healthy relationships are just a few others.

My big point here is that no matter how wonderful your diet, you can't expect to be at the peak of health if you don't exercise or sleep only four hours a night. So pick up those weights, get a good night's rest (and then another one, and another one), and stop worrying so much!

CHAPTER 9
Raw Food Success Stories

Well folks, that's it!

I've done my best to show you all the whys and hows of eating a low fat raw vegan diet. Hopefully you're now as convinced as I am that this way of eating, one that's focused on fresh and fruits and vegetables, is the greatest diet for health and vitality and you're now ready to put it to work in your own life.

If not, I've got one more trick up my sleeve. I'm going to turn it over to some wonderful individuals who have experienced amazing results since switching their diet to one focused on fresh fruits and vegetables.

Some eat all raw foods. Some eat mostly raw foods. All have an amazing story to share. Enjoy and prepare to be inspired!

"My skin glows and I look at least 5 years younger."

I started eating raw 6 months ago.

Before that I used to have constant gastritis and hereditary angioedema crisis (my bowels would swell to an excruciating pain taking me to hospitals at least once a month.) I suffered from insomnia every single night and had several manifestations of skin allergies.

All of those disappeared... I never had another angioedema crisis and my gastritis seem to be gone for good. My skin glows and I look at least 5 years younger. I look my best, I have this vibrant energy all day long and sleep like a child. I can see clearly what difference it made in my body and my mind. Eating a low-fat high carb, raw vegan diet was, by far, the best decision I ever made for my health.

Antonella Kalavati

"I feel like I could run forever if my body could handle it."

Both my wife and I started a vegan diet almost a year and a half ago. We stopped eating meat, dairy, eggs, and processed food. We try and maintain a mostly raw diet but do eat some cooked foods (no more than 20% of total calories). I myself have lost about 75 pounds and my wife has lost a little less. I am 60 years old, 5'10", and now weigh between 160-165.

I can't say what a life changing journey this has been. Even though I had no major medical problems, I've become so much healthier. The biggest improvement has been energy. I used to be a runner but I got so heavy I just couldn't do it anymore.

After about the first two weeks I noticed a big improvement in energy. As the weight began to come off I started running again. I just couldn't help it. I had so much energy and felt so good. I started out with just a couple of miles and worked my way up to four miles.

After talking to a friend of mine who was telling me how he was going to run in a half marathon (13 miles) I thought, "I can do that". So I started increasing the miles. No matter how far I went I was never out of breath. My cardiovascular function was off the charts.

I tried to be careful and not destroy my body by doing too much too soon, but I did. I hurt my knees and had to lay off for a while. I'm now running again but am keeping it to 4 miles 3 days a week. I feel like I could run forever if my body could handle it.

I also wake up earlier, and when I do, I'm energized and ready to get up. I'm no longer fuzzy headed and tired.

Larry Phillips

"People think I am crazy to eat so much fruit as a diabetic"

I recovered from a serious 15-year eating disorder 5 years ago. Part of my recovery process was asking God how to unselfishly nourish my body. Through a series of events and much research and trial and error, I found the low-fat/high-fruit raw vegan diet. Transitioning to this diet from my previous way of eating (worse than the standard American diet) has been extremely difficult, and quite a long process, but I am grateful beyond words to have found this unselfish—and extremely loving—way of eating.

I could go on and on, describing how my life has changed because of the low-fat raw vegan lifestyle. The most amazing parts for me, however, have to do with my chronic health conditions: type 1 diabetes and epilepsy.

When I first learned about all the health conditions from which people heal by eating raw foods, I felt I owed it a shot. Early on, I heard of someone going off their epilepsy medication.

My epilepsy has been termed "generalized seizure disorder", so I never had the every-day seizures that some people have. It was generally flashing/strobe lights, video games, lights flickering between trees while driving, and extremely low blood sugars that triggered my seizures—which were all-out "grand mal" seizures: lying on the floor, foaming at the mouth; seizures that freak other people out (not me, because I am unconscious during them; but I experience the after-effects of exhaustion, bruises and injuries from hitting things during my seizures, a chewed-up tongue, and the loss of driving privileges.)

When I had been eating raw a couple of months, I went off my epilepsy medication. When I told my neurologist what I had done, he tried to convince me to go back on medication, but when I refused, he told me that he couldn't see me anymore, and sent me a letter, documenting that I was going off medication "against medical advice". I didn't really know how long it took for things like epilepsy to heal, so I just was extremely careful to avoid situations that triggered seizures.

The one situation I had the most trouble avoiding was low blood sugars, as I was a soccer freak, and played for hours…which caused me to have very low blood sugars—very scary episodes. My strategy to avoid the low blood sugars was to set my blood sugar target range higher, and avoid going anywhere near a low blood sugar.

This did help to avoid lows, but it was terrible for my diabetes. Having higher blood sugars dramatically increases the risk for long-term diabetes complications, such as losing limbs, neuropathy, and blindness. I was terrified at the thought of getting complications, but didn't know what else to do.

I had experienced one low blood sugar seizure, about a year into eating raw foods, and definitely did not want to repeat that incident. But a dear friend (who has had a lot of health problems due to her own terrible blood sugar control) warned me that my blood sugars were really too high. I did some research and decided to take the risk and aim for lower blood sugars.

By the time I started working to lower my blood sugars, I had transitioned from high-fat raw to low-fat raw vegan. It had been about a year on low-fat raw vegan when I realized that I had experienced many extremely low blood sugars as a result of working to lower my overall blood sugar range, and that during this time, I had not had a single seizure! In the past, every time I experienced a very low blood sugar, I could count on a seizure. This was incredible to me—something is definitely changing in my body!

Another huge thing for me has been that I have succeeded in lowering my overall blood sugars—consistently—to the lowest I have ever had in my life! People think I am crazy to eat so much fruit as a diabetic, but I have documented over and over on my continuous glucose monitor that it is fat, not fruit sugar, that causes problems in my blood sugar control—again, amazing!

My diabetes doctor (who thought I was out of my mind to be eating so many carbs as a diabetic) was incredulous at my low basal insulin needs, my insulin: carbohydrate ratio, and my sensitivity to insulin. He still thinks there is no way my levels can be right because they are so low, even though he has been amazed at how my continuous glucose monitor readings looked like they could have been my husband's (without diabetes), and my lab results are so good.

And another HUGE thing for me is that 4 years ago, I went to my diabetic eye check-up at the ophthalmologist, and was told I had the beginnings of diabetic retinopathy. The next year at my visit, he told me there was a little more but it was still only the beginnings, so it didn't need surgery yet. When I moved and got a new ophthalmologist, he also saw the beginnings of retinopathy in my eyes at my yearly check-up.

However, THIS year when I went to see him (after about 1.5 years of mostly low-fat raw vegan), he said all traces of retinopathy in my left eye were now gone, and they had reduced from 3 micro-aneurysms to 1 in my right eye. It is reversing!!

Without going on and on forever, I will just say that so many health problems I created in my body through all the damage I did of over-exercising, under-resting, and over-eating massive amounts of junk are slowly reversing as I continue to attend to the basics of health: eating fresh fruits and lots of leafy greens, sleeping, getting sunshine, staying hydrated, etc.

Everything about my body is changing and getting healthier and feeling younger each day. I am grateful beyond words for those who have shared their experience and taught me how to live in a new way—going waaaay beyond surviving, to THRIVING.

Tasha Lee

Florida

HealthySkinnyBeautiful.com

"I hop out of bed in the morning as if I was a teenager"

Hi Swayze,

I have been on the raw food way of life for over 18 months now. The difference in my life has been astounding.

I lost 20kg of fat in 4 months in spite of eating huge amounts of delicious fresh fruit and vegetables. The great thing is that I don't have any lose skin! Even my eyelids and breasts got a lift. My skin is as tight as if I never had any weight issues.

The whites of my eyes are very white, my hair is a lot thicker, my sense of smell and taste are razor sharp now. "Foods" I used to like before like chips and biscuits hold no attraction to me whatsoever. Anything fried smells and tastes terrible to me.

My menopause symptoms like: hot flushes, mood sings and sweating went away within a couple of weeks of going raw and only come back if I have some cooked food occasionally (if we go out it sometimes is difficult to eat 100% raw).

Although I did not have any major illnesses before starting my journey, I had a lot of aches and pains, especially when getting up in the morning. All those - gone. I hop out of bed in the morning as if I was a teenager instead of being a grandma.

I feel so positive most of the time that I through out TV out of our bedroom because I cannot stand to watch the doom and gloom which is constantly delivered via tube. I feel happy and light.

Although physical changes gave been great, I find that the difference in my mind has been even greater. I used to be a couch potato all my life, now, suddenly I am beginning to do activities which were foreign to me. Things like: obstacle and high ropes course, riding a motorbike and going camping! Sometimes I do not recognize myself but darn it - I like the new me :-)

Victoria Winnard.

"My iron went up and now is at a normal level"

Hi Swayze,

My name is Lisa Marie Vasquez. I had serious iron issues since 2002 complete with dizzy spells and chronic fatigue. My ferritin was 4 (dangerously low). The doctors put me on iron pills 3 times a day, gave me a diet of red meat, liver, beans and spinach.

Finally I had surgery on Friday the 13th of 2009 to stop my periods because the doctors thought that will increase my ferritin count. It didn't work. They had no idea what to do with me. I dropped to my knees and prayed for help.

I bumped into a woman who was drinking green smoothies and asked her what it was. She shared with me how they helped her with depression. I asked her if they could help with low iron and she thought they could because they were made with greens. I tried that. Guess what - my iron went up and now is at a normal level.

Also in 2008 my HDL was 36, my cardiac risk ratio was 3.1 and my LDL was 59. In 2011 my HDL was 52 (doctors wanted in over 40), my cardiac risk ratio went down to 2.6 and my LDL is 57.

I thank the good Lord for the green smoothie, for raw foods, for helping to feel normal again.

Thanks for what you are doing to get this info out to people.

Much love and positive energy from Milwaukee.

Lisa

"I have lost 2kg...even though I am eating way more calories than before."

I am a keen runner and spend a fair amount of time swimming and on the spin bike, as well as working out at the gym. Over the last 7-8months, I have been battling many injuries from overtraining, as well as struggling with fatigue and massive food cravings, especially for sweet and salty food.

I struggled with my weight as well, despite a relatively huge training volume and watching what I eat. I was eating plenty of meat and whey protein, and relatively low fat and carbs.

My injuries, particularly my Achilles tendonitis and hamstring tendonitis, got so bad, I started hating exercise, especially running, which I used to love so much. I could hardly walk when I first got up in the mornings. As a physiotherapist, I tried everything possible to rehabilitate, but the pain remained.

I started reading many books on nutrition, and decided to turn to a LFRV [low fat raw vegan] diet. After being on it for 2 weeks, I no longer struggle with Achilles tendonitis, and my hamstring tendonitis is 70% better. I have taken 3 minutes off my 6km time, and could go faster except my dog was struggling to keep up with me.

I have lost 2kg, and my clothes are fitting me better, even though I am eating way more calories than before. I no longer crave bad food. Rather, I have started developing cravings for raw fruits and vegetables.

I was dubious when I first started out, but I was so desperate I would have given anything a go. I am now glad I did it, and am going to keep up with it.

Grace

"I'm 55 now, but I feel 20."

Hey Swayze,

Here is my story.....

I was overweight, around 170 lbs at 5'5", on Zocor (Zocor is used to lower cholesterol and triglycerides (types of fat) in the blood), and had breast cancer in 2006. I've also had eczema since I was 4 years old, but never could get rid of it. All the creams and steroids I took helped a little, but it would come back full force after stopping the drugs.

I had my 6 month blood test due in July of 2011 (to check on my cholesterol and liver panel). To my dismay, my liver enzymes were high. That scared me a lot. I had aches and muscle pain while taking the zocor, so I went online to find out what could be done.

I found some websites that mention raw foods to help lower cholesterol and lose weight. It was the high fat raw life way, so in August of 2011 I started my journey. By November my weight was down to 140 lbs which was amazing to me because I ate all I wanted without filling hungry.

In January or February I came upon your website and 30 bananas and learned about the low fat raw diet and how bad the high fat raw diet was for you. Since then I have lost more weight now 120 lbs at 5'5" small frame body. As an extra bonus my eczema has completely disappeared. I do have a red spot where it was, but no itching, scaling, or dryness.

I Love my fruit and my lb of greens, its just amazing to me I wish I had this knowledge when I was younger. I'm 55 now, but I feel 20. I have tons of energy...hehehe LOVE IT!!!!

Just wanted to say also that if I stray off this wonderful life style I get sick...nausea, palm of hands will break out into small blisters, itching will start where the ezcema was.

Ohh I almost forgot, my daughter now eats a lfrv [low fat raw vegan] diet and has lost 50 lbs and loves that she can eat and not starve while losing weight.

Hugs,

Annette

"Going raw has saved my life."

In The Beginning, there was no name to what I did. I simply moved through my day with a few simple goals: Don't eat. Look pretty. Be clever. And I did those three things all too well. By the end of high school I was thin, had long thick dark hair, big green eyes, clear skin, outstanding grades, and a future that everyone told me was promising. But still, I hated every last ounce of myself.

No number was good enough until it was perfect. And even then, it really never was that great. I had to get 100's on tests, I had to always jump higher and run further. I had to understand things faster than anyone else. I had to do ten more sit ups than yesterday, 100 less calories, one less pound, clean clear skin in the morning, a flat stomach in the showers, and ribs and bones and teeth and clothes and sizes and numbers and a crazed compulsion to be better than I ever was before.

At first there were no symptoms. At first the only issues were the ones violently and soundlessly waging war inside my own head. But soon enough I lost my period, lost my hair, broke my nails, and blacked out often. I was growing tired of my own games and this exhaustion and desperate hopelessness made me sloppy.

I stopped caring who saw how little I ate or how I obsessed over food. I kept journals of my torment in all too easily found places. These journals described horrible things and to this day I shudder at the thought of what my parents may have read. But they caught on quickly and intervened.

They took me places I didn't want to go—doctors and nutritionists and therapists. They did tests and asked me questions and I told them as much of the truth as I could. They in turn told me the things I already knew but didn't want to hear. I had an eating disorder, I had anorexia nervosa.

I was just beginning my freshman year of college and this diagnosis destroyed me. All of the sudden I had a disease. All of the sudden I needed to be fixed. All of the sudden I was weak and helpless and horrified. I was dying and it was more apparent each day.

My sides ached when I lay down to sleep, my vision blurred when I was too active, my butt fell asleep sitting on couches and chairs, my head spun when I stood up, I could hardly take baths for the pain of my spine and hip bones digging into the bottom of the tub, and masses of my hair washed away down the shower every morning. I was deficient in so many things and my bone density levels were low. I was at a higher risk of spinal fracture which could be induced by any activity more intense than walking.

And then there was the cold. It is actually indescribable unless you've felt it for yourself. A kind of violent constant chill wrapped around every inch of my body, it was an immobilizing sort of numb awful torture. It was the worst of all things bad.

So they tried to fix me their way. The doctor tried to give me medication. The therapist tried to pry open my thoughts and fix the reason why it all started. The nutritionist told me to eat more. I was vegetarian at the time and she consistently complained that I did not get enough protein in my diet. She advised masses of peanut butter, cheese, dairy and any other calorically dense fatty food—even fish! They must have wanted me to gain 30 pounds in about 2 months.

Clearly this kind of weight gain was not healthy and I somehow knew it. I struggled most of the winter, trying to up my calories and accept the fact that I would be fat again. But no matter how much I ate, I lost more weight. Nothing was helping and I was frightened.

Sooner or later I began to realize that the more fruits and vegetables I ate, the better I

felt. I started completely ignoring the nutritionist's advice and upping my calories with bananas or dates rather than peanut butter, nuts, seeds, cheese, eggs, and avocados that had given me acne, stomach discomfort, and gas.

I then remembered reading a blog post about a girl who was raw vegan. At the time when I had read it I had instantly fallen in love with the idea but knew I wasn't ready. But now I was. At the end of March I transitioned to a low fat raw vegan diet and it changed my life forever.

The fruity high you get when you first switch is like no other! You want to sing to the world about all the amazing wonders of fruit. It took all of my strength to keep from bursting with uncontrollable joy. I transitioned for a bit over a month and researched until my head hurt with all the information I stuffed into it. I would spend 3-5 hours every day reading everything I possibly could and watching videos on YouTube from the most inspiring and humorous people.

All this let me draw my own conclusions about why this diet was right for me.

The next time I had an appointment with the nutritionist she was appalled. Less than 10% of calories from fat and protein? Impossible! The medical doctor was horrified! She explained all the diseases and deficiency I could possibly obtain. Surely I would come down with an illness and never live to be 30! But wait, I had already done that.

This was me fixing that disease. It was a tough battle to win them over but in the consecutive months of blood tests and weight gain they realized that what I was doing was working for me—they just didn't know why.

Much to their disbelief, my protein, iron, and B12 levels always came back perfect, and I felt as amazing as I knew I was becoming. Over the summer I went from 100 pounds at 5'7.5" to 120 pounds where I stabilized. I could finally do everything I wanted and I finally felt amazing and happy all the awful voices left my head. There was no room for the negativity they thrived on.

The weight gain which would have once horrified me beyond any and all awfully imaginable things was suddenly perfectly acceptable because it came from the best food in the world. I knew that eating nothing but fresh ripe raw fruits, vegetables and a few nuts and seeds would automatically take me to my ideal weight and leave me there as happy as I could be. It will do it for anyone who gives this lifestyle an honest go.

I was still slim, but now I was healthy. I could love my body for what it was rather than hating it for what I had intentionally starved it to become.

Never once did I slip up and revert back to unhealthy cooked foods, let alone animal products. Becoming vegan for my health had the altogether most important side effect of becoming an ethical vegan. I obviously love animals and always have. But only after becoming vegan did I realize how much of a hypocrite I had been. How can one say they love animals, but then turn around and condone the needless torture and murder of animals so one can simply enjoy the taste of their dead flesh?

I now thrive on a low fat raw vegan diet. My digestion is perfect, I have no bodily odor, my skin has become clear once more, and I feel the amazing energy of this lifestyle every single day! I am finally happy.

Going raw has saved my life. It has completely cured me of my eating disorder. It has chased the horrible thoughts from my mind and taught me to value my body and the things my body tell me every day. It has saved my life and I am forever grateful.

Cortney

"My body is back to a healthy state both mentally and physically."

Hi,

I first started eating raw 9 months ago and love it.

I was very stressed and tired for a very long time and I just kept powering through till one day I couldn't cope anymore. It was making me depressed, I never wanted to do anything because it was all too much for me to cope with and after a visit to my Dr I had some tests done and I have a clump of cysts in my thyroid glands and my thyroid was over active, which basically meant I was burnt out.

The Dr advised to just monitor this over the months so over the next 6 months I kept going back in for my blood test and my results kept slipping and getting worst each time. This went on and over time I couldn't take it anymore so I did some research and put myself on a raw vegan diet as I did not want to be taking tablets for this condition.

After 3 months my test results stayed the same over 6 months my thyroid has gone back to being healthy to which I believe is all because of my diet. And I was able to fall pregnant naturally after a long time of trying. My body is back to a healthy state both mentally and physically.

Not only that, I feel amazing, my skin is amazing, my eyes are clear, my head is clear and I have so much more energy......

Good food makes me happy !

Regards,

Renee Coombs

"I went from laying around waiting to die to feeling great"

I started eating raw about 4 years ago, when I was very sick. I had extremely high blood pressure, my right ventricle of my heart was not functioning correctly and one of my eyes became blurred because of a vein that was cut off because of the high blood pressure.

So I went to the doctor and of course he gave me loads of drugs to take. I took them for a week and felt worse, horrible.

So I went to the library and researched things I could do besides drugs. I found a lot of good books and tried several ideas and diets. They seemed to help.

But then I went on the web and researched different diets looking for the perfect or best diet for humans. I discovered the raw diet, read several books and in no time, like about a month, I was feeling really good and my blood pressure was good and my eye sight improved, which the eye doctor said would never happen.

So from there with further and constant research I discovered 801010 diet and my health became amazing, better vision, perfect blood pressure, and perfect weight and unlimited energy.

So I went from laying around waiting to die to feeling great and working again and exercising everyday. And feeling like I discovered the fountain of youth! The raw diet is amazing!

Now I'm 52, but I feel like I'm in my twenties, the raw food diet changed my life and health. It really is the perfect human diet.

Thanks,

Nick

"Now my life doesn't revolve around food"

I absolutely love being on a raw food diet. It was difficult to get used to at first, but I decided in July 2011 that it was time for a drastic change.

I primarily ate high carb "vegetarian" meals which basically meant lots of noodles, breads and soups, cookies, cake, ice cream, nachos, cheese, just about anything that didn't look like it had meat in it. After tons of research, discussions with my doctor, and advice from friends and family, I decided to investigate a raw food diet.

Being a pseudo vegetarian wasn't as healthy as I thought. I had to face the facts at 22 years old I had bad knees, a bad back, constantly had irritated skin, and severe digestive problems which sometimes caused me to be backed up for over a week at a time.

Since starting a raw food diet, and slowly incorporating exercise into my life, I've not only lost over 70 pounds, but I have clear skin, strong and healthy hair and nails, my joints ache less, my visits to the chiropractor have lessened, my digestive system has become regular, and I haven't had a single illness, not even a little cold since last July.

Everything just started to feel better, I have more energy and I gained the will power to quit smoking and drinking. Now my life doesn't revolve around food, my body tells me I'm hungry and so I feed it to survive. It's an enlightening and empowering experience that I would recommend to anyone.

-Caitlin Barlow

24 years old

Boston, MA

"Now my nasal passages are so clear I can smell things a mile away."

Hi Swayze

Your email couldn't have come at a much better time.

I have been on this diet on and off since last year but about a month or two ago I decided to go 100% Raw. I can't explain the elation I'm feeling and the relief.

You see sinus & hay-fever issues have always been the story of my life. A few years ago my sister and I visited the E.N.T. So she goes first and the doc checks out her nose and says my dear your nasal passages are a pale pink you have the worst case of sinus. So I get a little worried and wonder what he has to say about me.

Then it's my turn and he barely checks out my nose when the look on his face surprises me. He goes OMW your case is even worse than your sister's. Your nasal passages aren't even pink, they're a pale blue. So you can only imagine how I must have been feeling. Scared, yes very. So I ask the doc how this can be solved and he says well you're allergic to preservatives which are pretty much in everything.

So I guess I won't be eating anything again. Or at least that's what I thought.

Then a couple of years later my GP diagnoses me with Fibromyalgia which is a chronic disease that affects the muscles at various points in the body. So I go home and google like crazy knowing doctors can easily misdiagnose this particular disease. Turns out he was wrong and I was actually suffering from carpal tunnel syndrome. So after I had searched the web hi & lo, near & far I found a solution and voila Raw Food was the only answer.

Yet still it took me a while to realize this.

Luckily I knew enough to go through both my pregnancies about 80-90% Raw. Thanks to that I now have 2 Gorgeously Little Love Monkeys who are crazy about their fruit & veggies. Even though they are only 4 and 2 they can finish a medium sized watermelon between themselves just for breakfast. Never mind the Green Smoothies, they love it to bits.

I must say all the fruits, veggies & nuts helps with their temperament. They are very busy boys but not hyper. We do crazy things like jumping on a trampoline, running around the park & we love the monkey bars. They are both very alert and very smart. Most say their mental development is above their age and that they way above their milestones. Because I've been home schooling them I was not aware of this. I just thought they were very bright, but didn't realize the extent. I truly base this on their diet.

Anyways enough about them let's get back to me.

Well this year after battling with my sinuses for 2 decades I decided to go Raw & after the first few days I could feel the difference as the mucous was being excreted via every orifice possible. I couldn't understand this but it all made sense in the end. Now my nasal passages are so clear I can smell things a mile away. Oh & my nasal passages are not only a pale pink but very pink. Haven't had any hay fever attacks for months now.

As for weight-loss I have released 9kg/20lbs in under 2 months. Of which I can tell you was fat-loss. I no longer have a muffin top or a jelly belly as my babies call it. My husband has even been eyeing me the way he did back when we first men when I was as thin as a bean pole. I still have about 13.5kgs/30lbs to release. I say release so it never comes back.

My hormones are finally in check. My period has even shortened going from a very uncomfortable, unbearable 7 days to the shortest 3 days of no pain or discomfort I've ever experienced in my life. You don't know how relieved and happy I am. This is the life people.

As for my emotions they no longer fluctuate. Its constant and I'm on a constant high and no I don't do any funny herbs or mushrooms. I'm naturally high on life.

I even got my mojo back and can't go a day without exercise or monkeying about with my Love Monkeys. I got my zest for life back. I thought I lost it all. Now I know who the culprit was that stole my joy. They are cousins called Cooked food and Junk food. I'm so glad they're no relative of mine. Not that they were, perhaps just acquaintances, but now I've cut them off completely. Kind of like a relationship gone bad. We've severed all ties or at least I have. Now my life is filled with Love, Joy, Peace & Happiness.

I feel so liberated and its reconnected my body, mind & spirit. I feel so connected to everyone and everything especially the beauty of our surroundings which we usually take for granted.

I hear this song and I just want to jump up and down "Release me by Agnes".

That's my getting over cooked food song. Just substitute person as cooked food.

So if you want to take back your life, reclaim your health first then everything else will fall into place.

Love Life, Live Life, Enjoy Life :)

Lotsa Fruity Love

Lee-Anne Lang

(Johannesburg, South Africa)

"I have dropped 50 pounds and feel very much better."

Swayze;

I am 59 years old and have been overweight most all of my life. Six months ago I found your website and became very interested in what you have to say. I am an educated person (an attorney) and have always been very interested in how the body works. I have studied on my own about nutrition and health. Eating raw fruits and vegetables makes sense to me. I still try to read everything I can about nutrition and eating raw.

I have been about 90% raw for six months. I hope to become total raw soon. I have dropped 50 pounds and feel very much better. I have more energy and a much more positive outlook. While I have quite a ways to go still (about 100 more pounds) I believe that eating raw fruits and vegetables is definitely going to get me to my ideal weight and contribute to a much longer, healthier and happier life.

Thank you so much for what you do.

Sincerely,

Charles Thorn

"I have been able to reduce my medication TWICE!!"

Hi Swayze,

First of all thank you so much for all your supportive emails, they (and you) are truly inspirational.

Just a little bit about myself - I live on a tiny Island in the middle of the Irish Sea (Isle of Man). I was diagnosed with an under active thyroid over 10 years ago and have been on the same dose of medication until I started eating a low fat, high fruit diet about 12 months ago. Since that time, I have been able to reduce my medication TWICE!! Something I couldn't even consider during the past 10 years.

Also, during the last 12 months, I started with symptoms of menopause, predominantly night sweats which were horrendous and resulted in loss of sleep for many, many nights. Eating raw and introducing Maca into my diet saw the sweats disappear almost overnight. My doctor couldn't believe it - indeed one "lady doctor" in the surgery advised me that the only thing for menopausal sweats was HRT - obviously I didn't take her advice.

Eating raw is becoming a way of life to me and it has changed my life completely. My energy levels are through the roof - I am a grandmother and I will be 55 years old in 10 days and I attend bootcamp 4 days a week at 6am and I am the oldest member - my daughter runs it and they call me the "Mummy Machine" which I take as a compliment. I want to carry on as long as possible with my exercise because I absolutely love it.

I want to keep learning as much as I can about raw food and I have met some wonderful people on my journey. I feel so blessed.

Once again Swayze keep up the good word. None of this would have been possible for me without people like you. You motivate me and inspire me.

Thank you so much.

Love and blessings

Linda

xxx :-)

"Eating a high raw, high fruit, low fat vegan diet is, for me, a life saver."

Hi Swayze

In 2009 I was finally diagnosed with histaminosis (a severe form of histamine intolerance), some kind of reactive arthritis and mast cell activation syndrome. For years I had been having different bouts of symptoms as I reacted to common chemicals such as toothpaste, face cream, body lotion and household cleaning products. The smell of perfume could send me into shock with breathing difficulties, sweating, .. the whole works.

I also reacted adversely to antihistamines and other medications. I fell asleep suddenly after eating certain foods and in air-conditioned places such as on trains and planes and often could not be woken up (so much so I was robbed on several occasions while I slept!).

I felt like I was getting sicker each day. I had joint pain, frequent soreness of skin and scalp, my hair was falling out and I had to stop using hair dye and finally I shaved my head as the touch of my dyed hair on my skin caused big weals to appear.

I had frequent choking sessions especially while asleep at night as my body would go into a sort of anaphylaxis (I was told it was not sleep apnoea). I also had skin problems such as rashes and hives; headaches, severe diarrhoea, weight gain, the list went on and on. My anxiety levels were sky high as you might imagine.

To cut a long story short, after consulting a lot of doctors to no avail, I met a biochemist (who was specializing in the immune system and histamine issues) who did a lot of tests and told me the bad news … He also told me that I had to change my diet and lifestyle radically to have a chance of stopping the choking bouts etc which were becoming so severe. He recommended that I try raw, low histamine food.

I did a lot of research and found the raw food diet. I also found there were several different versions, gourmet raw, high fat, etc. Of course I made many mistakes trying to find the optimum diet for me. I had to cut out all fermented foods and I found that the higher fat gourmet raw type of diet did not work for me. I started writing a blog called The Reluctant Raw Foodist. I called myself that as I was forced by my health issues to change my diet and I found it very hard at first.

I now follow a high raw, high fruit, low fat vegan diet including lots of greens and I am feeling better and better. My skin rashes are gone, my night choking is gone, I have lost weight and I am starting to be able to tolerate perfumes enough to go to the theatre and to travel on trains again. I have not tried going on a plane yet. I still have a stressful life as my mother has dementia and my husband has to have daily care following a stroke but my anxiety levels are well down and I feel much more able to cope. Eating a high raw, high fruit, low fat vegan diet is, for me, a life saver.

Thank you so much for your useful and practical tips and advice. I have consulted your website a lot over the last couple of years.

Su
aka The Reluctant Raw Foodist

http://www.thereluctantrawfoodist.com

"I was on four prescription drugs and now I am drug free"

My name is Judy and I am a 64 year old wife, mother, retired school teacher, friend, yoga lover and generally a compulsive person. I have been 100 percent 80/10/10 for almost 5 years. When I started this journey I was compulsive eating on four prescription drugs and not feeling very energetic or healthy.

I went to a talk in Michigan by Ellen Livingston, bought Doug Graham's book and Don Bennett's book, read them and went raw the next day. I also took a class from Ellen in her home that helped me fine tune my journey. It has been an incredible journey to a more healthy me physically, emotionally and spiritually. G-d is good and I am blessed.

Well Swayze you want to know some results over the years. I have been so healthy there hasn't been a need to go for my yearly physical. I just don't get sick. I have more energy than most 20 year olds I know. I do go to the dentist twice a year and the dental hygienist is amazed at how healthy my gums and mouth are and wants to know what I do.

I had psoriasis but now it is gone. I was on four prescription drugs and now I am drug free except for taking a B 12 and Vitamin D3 when I remember. Maybe once a week or once a month. LOL My age spots on my face have disappeared or lightened. When people find out how old I am they are amazed and say they don't believe it.

I feel I am a kinder more loving person. I am more accepting of others. I still cook and bake for my husband, family and friends. I just pray over their food and put my love into it. Of course my son says I use to be an amazing cook and now I am not as good because I won't taste the food. It is not mine and it doesn't interest me. Sometimes the smell will bring back an awesome memory and I can just relish in the memory.

Although I cook for family and friends I always start the meal with a table full of fruit and vegetables for everyone to munch on before I serve dinner. Then I serve a big salad or two with dinner along with a raw desert and a SAD [standard American diet] desert. I love my food and can't even imagine eating any other way. I now wear out my clothes and have been wearing a size four for years now, an amazing difference from my size 22. Hmm mm Any other results.....Can't think of any at the moment... I am blessed and life is good.

Take care and be good to yourself Swayze. Enjoy! Happy Holidays!

With love and peace,

Judy

"I am now free of colds, allergies, skin rashes, aches and pains"

Swayze,

I remember the days of running from fast food drive thru to drive thru eating whatever supersized meal that came wrapped in a decorative logo-paper and wondering why I never felt all that great on the "food" that supposedly we were "meant to eat". It wasn't until I had an emergency appendectomy that I decided to, not only change my diet, but also to find out what the true human diet was supposed to be.

I started by reading Harvey and Marilyn Diamond's classic diet book "Fit for Life" and never turned back after that. I went from healthy "meats" and low fat milk, to vegetarian, to vegan, to gourmet raw and finally, after reading Dr. Graham's 80/10/10 diet book, settled on low fat raw. I went about 95% raw for 5 years (I still eat steamed potatoes or other cruciferous veggies) and I have been 100% LFR for the past 2 years.

It has been so helpful to discover the great information that people, like Frederic Patenaude, Kevin Gianni and of course you, Swayze Foster, have been writing on the internet and this is such a boost to staying on this raw adventure.

It has taken a while but I am now free of colds, allergies, skin rashes, aches and pains and I have almost boundless energy which is commented on constantly by friends and co-workers. I see this same pattern with everyone I know who is following this diet. For me the raw lifestyle has been a godsend! I would never go back to non-vegan cooked lifeless foods.

When I started this diet journey there were not many resources out there to assist in the transition to a healthier way of living. Because of people like you we now have some much needed help. I have really relied on your recipe book and also your book on ending the cravings I had for cooked food. I believe that the low fat raw diet can make noticeable improvements in anyone's life and certainly your information makes it just that much easier to follow.

Keep up the positive reinforcement!!

Bill Kranker

"I don't need to sleep as much and still feel rested when I wake up on the morning."

I came to eating a low fat, high fruit raw food diet after already being vegan/macrobiotic and raw vegan (but not low fat) for over 18 years. I have never had any health issues, per se, but I have seen some great results from eating this way that perhaps others have never paid attention to.

My cycle is much shorter, lighter with no pain like I had when I first became vegan over 20 years ago. I eliminate many times a day and it doesn't take me much time in the bathroom (this is an important part in telling the health of your body). I don't need to sleep as much and still feel rested when I wake up on the morning. My mind has become sharper and clearer, in the sense that I can retain information and also figure out the solutions easily- there is no cloudiness/forgetfulness.

These may not seem as "BIG" as serious dis-eases, but they are important because most people had/have experienced these things and don't see any relationship/connection with the food they consume on a daily basis. Everything is cumulative and in time will have an affect on your physical body (as well as how you feel emotionally, socially, psychologically).

It is important because if you can eliminate these mild issues mostly through your food choices you will not likely have to ever deal with debilitating health conditions in the future (along with all the stress that comes with it - financial costs, visiting doctors and hospitals, taking medications that usually have side affects, etc). It is better to prevent it to begin with. Choosing to eat low fat, high fruit raw vegan is a great first step in the right direction for achieving optimal health and wellness.

Chef Mindy

rawsomegal.wordpress.com

"We've found the fountain of youth, and we're sticking to it."

Eating low fat, vegan, raw food allowed me to easily release 42 lbs (and counting), and my husband lost 24 lbs. He's back to his high school weight and wearing a 32 inch waist from a 36. I've gone from a size 22 to a 14.

We also completely eliminated our daily heartburn. I'm 46 and my husband is 56, and we feel 20 years younger in terms of our energy. Being empty nesters it's like we're on our honeymoon again!

We've found the fountain of youth, and we're sticking to it. My husband had high cholesterol, over 200 and now it's only 145, and he no longer snores. For the first time in my life, I have no doubts about how I'll lose the rest of my weight. I don't even worry about it anymore, or give it much thought because low fat, vegan and raw, is the answer.

Stephanie L. Watson

Conclusion

In the introduction to this book, I asked if you were ready. I asked if you were ready to go raw so you can experience the best body, energy, digestion, and overall well-being of your life.

So are you?

Are you ready to eat a diet that's comprised of the most nutritious, delicious, and satisfying foods on the planet?

Are you ready to eat a diet with the power to protect you from heart disease, stroke, diabetes, cancer, and other diseases and disorders?

Are you ready to eat a diet with the power to protect you from colds, flus, allergies, migraines, and joint pains?

Are you ready to eat a diet with the power to bring you tons of energy and mental clarity without coffee, sodas, energy drinks, or other unhealthy stimulants?

Are you ready to eat a diet with the power to release excess fat and help you reach your ideal weight, not for the next few years, but for the rest of your life?

Yes? Then get to it!

I've shown you what it takes to do the raw food diet right. Now it's your turn to put it into practice.

Don't worry, that doesn't mean eating all raw right now. In fact, I don't recommend that. It simply means getting started.

A really simple way to get started is to make one meal a day raw. Breakfast works for many people. Have a melon or a few mangoes or a delicious green smoothie. The possibilities are endless. (Make sure to refer back to the sample meal plan in chapter five for more ideas.)

If that seems too difficult right now, try three meals a week raw or even just one meal a week! It doesn't matter how you transition (or how long you take) as long as it's a stress-free plan that works for you. (Stressing out about food is not good stress!)

If you'd like more transitioning tips, be sure to check out this book's companion video "Simple Tips for Raw Food Success" at *www.scienceofraw.com/success*

Also, be sure to check out the Fit On Raw blog (*www.fitonraw.com/blog*) where you'll find over 350 free articles and videos all about thriving on a raw food lifestyle.

Now, wonderful reader, it's time to say goodbye. I truly hope this book has educated, motivated, and inspired you to eat a diet focused on the freshest, tastiest, healthiest foods on the planet: fresh fruits and vegetables.

Go raw and be fit,

Swayze Foster

References

Chapter 1: Why Vegan?

1.   Campbell, C. T., & Campbell, T. M. (2006). *The China Study: Starling Implications for Diet, Weight Loss and Long-Term Health.* Dallas, TX: BenBella Books.

2.   Esselstyn, Caldwell B. Jr. (2007). *Prevent and Reverse Heart Disease: The Revolutionary, Scientifically Proven, Nutrition-Based Cure.* New York, NY: Penguin Group.

3.   Dalessandri K.M., & Organ C.H. Jr. (1995). Surgery, drugs, lifestyle, and hyperlipidemia. *Am J Surg*, 169(4):374-378.

4.   Prospective Studies Collaboration, Lewington S., Whitlock G., Clarke R., Sherliker P., Emberson J., . . . Collins R. (2007). Blood cholesterol and vascular mortality by age, sex, blood pressure: a meta-analysis of individual data from 61 prospective studies with 55,000 vascular deaths. *Lancet*, 370(9602):1829-1839.

5.   Framingham Heart Study. Research Milestones. Retrieved from ***http://www.framinghamheartstudy.org/about/milestones.html***

6.   American College of Cardiology (2012). Lowering LDL, the earlier the better. *ScienceDaily*. Retrieved from ***http://www.sciencedaily.com/releases/2012/03/120326133606.htm***

7.   Murphy, S.L., Xu, J., Kochanek, K.D., Division of Vital Statistics (2012). Deaths: preliminary Data for 2010. *National Vital Statistics Reports*, 60(4). Retrieved from ***http://www.cdc.gov/nchs/data/nvsr/nvsr60/nvsr60_04.pdf***

8.   Fuhrman, J. (2003). *Eat To Live: The Revolutionary Formula for Fast and Sustained Weight Loss.* New York, NY: Little, Brown and Company.

9.   McDougall, J.A. High Cholesterol. Retrieved from ***http://www.drmcdougall.com/med_cholesterol.html***

10.   Furie, K.L., Kasner, S.E., Adams, R.J., Albers, G.W., Bush, R.L., Fagan, S.C., … Interdisciplinary Council on Quality of Care and Outcomes Research (2011). Guidelines for the Prevention of Stroke in Patients With Stroke or Transient Ischemic Attack. *AHA/ASA Guideline*, 42:227-276.

11.   Swinburn, B.A., Metcalf, P.A., Ley, S.J. (2001). Long-Term (5-Year) Effects of a Reduced-Fat Diet Intervention in Individuals With Glucose Intolerance. *Diabetes Care*, 24:619-624.

12.   University of North Carolina School of Medicine (2011). Link between high-fat diet and type 2 diabetes clarified. *ScienceDaily*. Retrieved from ***http://www.sciencedaily.com/releases/2011/04/110411121539.htm***

13.   Sieri, S., Krogh, V., Ferrari, P., Berrino, F., Pala, V., Thiébaut, A.C.M., … Riboli, E. (2008). Dietary fat and breast cancer risk in the European Prospective Investigation into Cancer and Nutrition. *Am J Clin Nutr*, 88(5):1304-1312.

14.   Llaverias, G., Danilo, C., Mercier, I., Daumer, K., Capozza, F., Williams, T.M., … Frank, P.G. (2010). Role of Cholesterol in the Development and Progression of Breast Cancer. *The American Journal of Pathology*, 178(1):402-412.

15.   Thiébaut, A.C.M., Kipnis, V., Chang, S., Subar, A.F., Thompson, F.E., Rosenberg, P.S., … Schatzkin, A. (2007). Dietary Fat and Postmenopausal Invasive Breast Cancer in the National Institutes of Health—AARP Diet and Health Study Cohort. *JNCI J Natl Cancer Inst*, 99(6):451-462.

16.   Qadir, M.I., & Malik, S.A. (2008). Plasma lipid profile in gynecologic cancers. *Eur J Gynaecol Oncol.*, 29(2):158-161.

17.   de Wit N., Derrien M., Bosch-Vermeulen, H., Oosterink, E., Keshtkar, S., Duval, C., … van der Meer, R. (2012). Saturated fat

stimulates obesity and hepatic steatosis and affects gut microbiota composition by an enhanced overflow of dietary fat to the distal intestine. *Am J Physiol Gastriointest Liver Physiol.*, 303(5):589-599.

18.   Phillips, C.M., Kesse-Guyot, E., McManus R., Hercberg, S., Lairon, D., Planells, R., & Roche, H.M. High dietary saturated fat intake accentuates obesity risk associated with the fat mass and obesity-associated gene in adults. *J Nutr.*, 142(5):824-831.

19.   Helzlsouer, K.J., Alberg, A.J., Norkus, E.P., Morris, J.S., Hoffman, S.C., & Comstock, G.W. (1996). Prospective Study of Serum Micronutrients and Ovarian Cancer. *J Natl Cancer Inst*, 88:32-37.

20.   Tania, M., Khan, M.A., & Song, Y. (2010). Association of lipid metabolism with ovarian cancer. *Curr Oncol.*, 17(5):6-11.

21.   Huncharek, M., Kupelnick, B. (2001). Dietary fat intake and risk of epithelial ovarian cancer: a meta-analysis of 6,689 subjects from 8 observational studies. *Nutr Cancer*, 40(2):87-91.

22.   European Society for Medical Oncology (2006). Direct Link Between High Cholesterol And Prostate Cancer Found. *ScienceDaily*. Retrieved from ***http://www.sciencedaily.com/releases/2006/04/060411231430.htm***

23.   Shafique, K., McLoone, P., Qureshi, K., Leung, H., Kart, C., & Morrison, D.S. (2012). Cholesterol and the risk of grade-specific prostate cancer incidence: evidence from two large prospective cohort studies with up to 37 years' follow up. *BMC Cancer*, 12:25.

24.   UroToday (2008). Diet High In Saturated Fat Contributes To Prostate Cancer Treatment Failure, Study Suggests. *ScienceDaily*. Retrieved from ***http://www.sciencedaily.com/releases/2008/05/080508184143.htm***

25.   Whittemore, A.S., Kolonel, L.N., Wu, A.H., John, E.M., Gallagher, R.P., Howe, G.R., ... et al. (1995). Prostate cancer in relation to diet, physical activity, and body size in blacks, whites, and

Asians in the United States and Canada. *J Natl Cancer Inst*, 87(9):652-661.

26.   Järvinen, R., Knekt, P., Hakulinen, T., Rissanen, H., & Heliövaara, M. (2001). Dietary fat, cholesterol and colorectal cancer in a prospective study. *Br J Cancer*, 8593:357-361.

27.   Cross, A.J., Leitzmann, M.F., Subar, A.F., Thompson, F.E., Hollenbeck, A.R., Schatzkin, A. (2009). A Prospective study of Meat and Fat Intake in Relation to Small Intestinal Cancer. *Cancer Res*, 68(22):9274-9279.

28.   Brigham and Women's Hospital (2012). With fat: What's good or bad for the heart, may be the same for the brain. *ScienceDaily*. Retrieved from ***http://www.sciencedaily.com/releases/2012/05/120518081358.htm***

29.   Baer, H.J., Glynn, R.J., Hu, F.B., Hankinson, S.E., Willett, W.C., Colditz, G.A., ... Rosner, B. (2011). Risk Factors for Mortality in the Nurses' Health Study: A Competing Risks Analysis. *Am J Epidemiol*, 173(3):319-329.

30.   Vergnaud, A., Norat, T., Romaguera, D., Mouw, T., May, A.M., Travier, N., ... Peeters, P.H.M. (2010). Meat consumption and prospective weight change in participants of the EPIC-PANACEA study. *Am J Clin Nutr*, 92(2):398-407.

31.   Griffin, R.M. (2010). How Fiber Helps Your Digestive Health. *WebMD*. Retrieved from ***http://www.webmd.com/diet/fiber-health-benefits-11/fiber-digestion?***

32.   Burton-Freeman, B. (2000). Dietary Fiber and Energy Regulation. *J Nutr*, 130(2S Suppl):272S-275S.

33.   Arora, T., Sharma R., & Frost, G. (2011). Propionate. Anti-Obesity and satiety enhancing factor? *Appetite*, 56(2):511-515.

34.   Hippe, B., Zwielehner, J., Liszt, K., Lassl, C., Unger, F., & Haslberger, A.G. (2011). Quantification of butyryl CoA:acetate

CoA-transferase genes reveals different butyrate production capacity in individuals according to diet and age. *FEMS Microbiology Letters*, 316(2):130-135.

35.   Brewer, G.J. (2009). The Risks of Copper Toxicity Contributing to Cognitive Decline in the Aging Population and to Alzheimer's Disease. *J Am Coll Nutr*, 28(3):238-242.

36.   Morris, M.C., Evans, D.A., Bienias, J.L. Tangney, C.C., Bennett, D.A., Aggarwal, N., ... Wilson, R.S. (2003). Dietary fats and the risk of incident Alzheimer disease. *Arch Neurol*, 60(2):194-200.

37.   de Batlle, J., Mendez, M., Romieu, I., Balcells, E., Benet, M., Donaire-Gonzalez, D., ... PAC-COPD Study Group (2012). Cured meat consumption increases risk of readmission in COPD patients. *ERJ*, 40(3):555-560.

38.   Jiang, R., Paik, D.C., Hankinson, J.L., & Barr, G. (2007). Cure Meat Consumption, Lung Function, and Chronic Obstructive Pulmonary Disease among United States Adults. *Am. J. Respir. Crit. Care Med*, 175(8):798-804.

39.   Jiang, R., Camargo, C.A. Jr, Varraso, R., Paik, D.C., Willett, W.C., & Barr, G.R. (2008). Consumption of cured meats and prospective risk of chronic obstructive pulmonary disease in women. *Am J Clin Nutr*, 87(4):1002-1008.

40.   Varraso, R., Fung, T.T., Barr, G.R., Hu, F.B., Willett, W., & Camargo, C.A. Jr. (2007). Prospective study of dietary patterns and chronic obstructive pulmonary disease among US women. *Am J Clin Nutr*, 86(2):488-495.

41.   Giem, P., Beeson, W.L., & Fraser, G.E. (1993). The incidence of dementia and intake of animal products: preliminary from the Adventist Health Study. *Neuroepidemiology*, 12(1):28-36.

42.   Albanese, E., Dangour, A.D., Uauy, R., Acosta, D., Guerra, M., Gallardo Guerra, S.S., ... Prince, M.J. (2009). Dietary fish and meat intake and dementia in Latin America, China, and India: a 10/66

Dementia Research Group population-based study. *Am J Clin Nutr*, 90(2):392-400.

43.   Ghanim, H., Abuaysheh, S., Sia, C.L., Korzeniewski, K., Chaudhuri, A., Fernandez-Real, J.M., & Dandona, P. (2009). Increase in Plasma Endotoxin Concentrations and the Expression of Toll-Like Receptors and Suppressor of Cytokine Signaling-3 in Mononuclear Cells After a High-Fat, High-Carbohydrate Meal. *Diabetes Care*, 32(12):2281-2287.

44.   Harte, A.L., Varma, M.C., Tripathi, G., McGee, K.C., Al-Daghri, Al-Attas, O.S., ... McTernan, P.G. (2012). High fat intake leads to acute postprandial exposure to circulating endotoxin in type 2 diabetic subjects. *Diabetes Care*, 35(2):375-382.

45.   González, C.A., Jakszyn, P., Pera, G., Agudo, A., Bingham, S., Palli, D., ... Riboli, E (2006). Meat Intake and Risk of Stomach and Esophageal Adenocarcinoma Within the European Prospective Investigation Into Cancer and Nutrition. *JNCI J Natl Cancer Inst*, 98(5):345-354.

46.   Keszei, A.P., Schouten, L.J., Goldbohm, R.A., & van den Brandt, P.A. (2012). Red and processed meat consumption and the risk of esophageal and gastric cancer subtypes in The Netherlands Cohort Study. *Ann Oncol*, 23(9):2319-2326.

47.   Cross, A.J., Leitzmann, M.F., Gail, M.H., Hollenbeck, A.R., Schatzkin, A., & Sinha, R. (2007). A Prospective Study of Red and Processed Meat Intake in Relation to Cancer Risk. *PLoS Med*, 4(12):e325.

48.   Choi, H.K., Mount, D.B., & Reginato, A.M. (2005). Pathogenesis of Gout. *Ann Intern Med*, 143(7):499-516.

49.   Reddy, S.T., Wang, C.Y., Sakhaee, K., Brinkley, L., & Pak, C.Y. (2002). Effect of low-carbohydrate high-protein diets on acid-base balance stone-forming propensity, and calcium metabolism. *Am J Kidney Dis*, 40(2):265-274.

50.   Breslau, N.A., Brinkley, L., Hill, K.D., & Pak, C.Y. (1988) Relationship of animal protein-rich diet to kidney stone formation and calcium metabolism. *J Clin Endocrinol Metab, 66(1)*:140-146.

51.   Freedman, N.D., Cross, A.J., McGlynn, K.A., Abnet, C.C., Park, Y., Hollenbeck, A.R., ... Sinha, R. (2010). Association of Meat and Fat Intake With Liver Disease and Hepatocellular Carcinoma in the NIH-AARP Cohort. *J Natl Cancer Inst*, 102(17):1354-1365.

52.   Campbell, W.W., & Tang, M. (2010). Protein Intake, Weight Loss, and Bone Mineral Density in Postmenopausal Women. *J Gerontol A Biol Med Sci*, 65A(10):1115-1122.

53.   Okubo, H., Sasaki, S, Horiguchi, H., Oguma, E., Miyamoto, K., Hosoi, Y., ... Kayama, F. (2006). Dietary patterns associated with bone mineral density in premenopausal Japanese farmwomen. *Am J Clin Nutr*, 83(5):1185-1192.

54.   Peters, J.M., Preston-Martin, S., London, S.J., Bowman, J.D., Buckley, J.D., & Thomas, D.C. (1994). Processed meats and risk of childhood leukemia (California, USA). *Cancer Causes Control*, 5(2):195-202.

55.   Liu, C.Y., Hsu, Y.H., Wu, M.T., Pan, P.C., Ho, C.K., Su, L., ... Kaohsiung Leukemia Research Group (2009). Cured meat, vegetables, and bean-curd foods in relation to childhood acute leukemia risk: a population based case-control study. *BMC Cancer*, 9:15.

56.   Stolzenberg-Solomon, R.Z., Cross, A.J., Silverman, D.T., Schairer, C., Thompson, F.E., Kipnis, V., ... Sinha, R. (2007). Meat and meat-mutagen intake and pancreatic cancer risk in the NIH-AARP cohort. *Cancer Epidemiol Biomarkers Prev*, 16(12):2664-2675.

57.   Anderson, K.E., Mongin, S.J., Sinha, R., Stolzenberg-Solomon, R., Gross, M.D., Ziegler, R.G., ... Church, T.R. (2012). Pancreatic cancer risk: associations with meat-derived carcinogen intake in the Prostate, Lung, Colorectal and Ovarian Cancer Screening Trial (PLCO) cohort. *Mol Carcinog*, 51(1):128-137.

58.   Kutlu, A., Oztürk, S., Taşkapan, O., Onem, Y., Kiralp, M.Z., & Ozçakar, L. (2010). Meat-induced joint attacks, or meat attacks the joint: rheumatism versus allergy. Nutr Clin Pract, 25(1):90-91.

59.   John Wiley & Sons, Inc. (2004). Eating Red Meat May Increase The Risk Of Rheumatoid Arthritis. *ScienceDaily*. Retrieved from ***http://www.sciencedaily.com/releases/2004/12/041203092152.htm***

60.   Larsson, S.C., Bergkvist, L., & Wolk, A. (2006). Processed meat consumption, dietary nitrosamines and stomach cancer risk in a cohort of Swedish women. *Int J Cancer*, 119(4):915-919.

61.   De Stefani, E., Ronco, A., Brennan, P., & Boffetta, P. (2001). Meat consumption and risk of stomach cancer in Uruguay: a case-control study. *Nutr Cancer*, 40(2):103-107.

62.   Palli, D., Russo, A., Ottini, L., Masala, G., Saieva, C., Amorosi, A., … Fraumeni, F.J. Jr. (2001). Red meat, family history, and increased risk of gastric cancer with microsatellite instability. *Cancer Res*, 61(14):5415-5419.

63.   Muntoni, S., Cocco, P., Aru, G., & Cucca, F. (2000). Nutritional factors and worldwide incidence of childhood type 1 diabetes. *Am J Clin Nutr*, 71(6):1525-1529.

64.   Bushinsky, D.A., Smith, S.B., Gavrilov, K.L., Gavrilov, L.F., Li, J, & Levi-Setti, R. (2003). Chronic acidosis-induced alteration in bone bicarbonate and phosphate. *Am J Physiol Renal Physiol*, 285(3):F532-539.

65.   Wiederkehr, M., & Krapf, R. (2001). Metabolic and endocrine effects of metabolic acidosis in humans. *Swiss Med Wkly*, 131(9-10):127-132.

66.   Dawson-Hughes, B., Harris, S.S., & Ceglia, L. (2008). Alkaline diets favor lean tissue mass in older adults. *Am J Clin Nutr*, 87(3):662-665.

67.   FoodSafety.gov. Bacteria and Viruses. Retrieved from *http://www.foodsafety.gov/poisoning/causes/bacteriaviruses/index.html*

68.   Johnson, J.R., Kuskowski, M.A., Smith, K., O-Bryan, T.T., & Tatini, S. (2005). Antimicrobial-resistant and extraintestinal pathogenic Escherichia coli in retail foods. *J Infect Dis*, 191(7):1040-1049.

69.   Sinha, R., Kuldorff, M., Chow, W.H., Denobile, J., & Rothman, N. (2001). Dietary intake of heterocyclic amines, meat-derived mutagenic activity, and risk of colorectal adenomas. *Cancer Epidemiol Biomarkers Prev*, 10(5):559-562.

70.   Butler, L.M., Sinha, R., Millikan, R.C., Martin, C.F., Newman, B., Gammon, M.D., ... Sandler, R.S. (2003). Heterocyclic Amines, Meat Intake, and Association with Colon Cancer in a Population-based Study. *Am J Epidemiol*, 157(5):434-445.

71.   Phillips, D.H. (1999). Polycyclic aromatic hydrocarbons in the diet. *Mutat Res*, 443(1-2):139-147.

72.   Tasevska, N., Sinha, R., Kipnis, V, Subar, A.F., Leitzmann, M.F., Hollenbeck, A.R., ... Cross, A.J. (2009). A prospective study of meat, cooking methods, meat mutagens, heme iron, and lung cancer risks. *Am J Clin Nutr*, 89(6):1884-1894.

73.   Goldberg, T., Cai, W., Peppa, M., Dardaine, V., Baliga, B.S., Uribarri, J., & Vlassara H. (2004). Advanced glycoxidation end products in commonly consumed foods. *J Am Diet Assoc*, 104(8):1287-1291.

74.   Uribarri, J., & Tuttle, K.R. (2006). Advanced glycation end products and nephrotoxicity of high-protein diets. *Clin J Soc Nephrol*, 1(6):1293-1299.

75.   Loglisci, R. (2010, Dec 23). New FDA Numbers Reveal Food Animals Consume Lion's Share of Antibiotics. Retrieved from *http://www.livablefutureblog.com/2010/12/new-fda-numbers-reveal-food-animals-consume-lion%E2%80%99s-share-of-antibiotics*

76.   The Economic Times (2012, Feb 1). How superbugs become resistant to antibiotics. Retrieved from *http://articles.economictimes.indiatimes.com/2012-02-01/news/31013009_1_superbugs-bacteria-enzymes*

77.   Avila, J. (2012, Jul 11). REPORT: Superbug Dangers in Chicken Linked to 8 Million At-Risk Women. ABC News. Retrieved from *http://abcnews.go.com/blogs/health/2012/07/11/superbug-dangers-in-chicken-linked-to-8-million-at-risk-women/*

78.   Grush, L. (2012, Sep 18). Deadly 'superbugs' on the rise: What you need to know. FoxNews.com. Retrieved from *http://www.foxnews.com/health/2012/09/18/deadly-uperbugs-on-rise-what-need-to-know/*

79.   University of Illinois at Urbana-Champaign (2007). Team Tracks Antibiotic Resistance From Swine Farms to Groundwater. *ScienceDaily*. Retrieved from *http://www.sciencedaily.com/releases/2007/08/070821153926.htm*

80.   University of Iowa (2012). High levels of MRSA bacteria in U.S. retail meat products, study suggests. *ScienceDaily*. Retrieved from *http://www.sciencedaily.com/releases/2012/01/120120182427.htm*

81.   Adams, J.U. (2012, Jan 30). Antibiotic-Free Meat Not Free of Drug-Resistant Bacteria. *ScienceMag*. Retrieved from *http://news.sciencemag.org/sciencenow/2012/01/organic-meat-not-free-of-drug-re.html*

82.   Gray, J., Nudelman, J., & Engel, C. (2010). State of the Evidence: The Connection Between Breast Cancer and the Environment. Breast Cancer Fund. Retrieved from *http://www.breastcancerfund.org/assets/pdfs/publications/state-of-the-evidence-2010.pdf*

83.   World Health Organization (2010). Dioxins and their effects on human health. Retrieved from *http://www.who.int/mediacentre/factsheets/fs225/en/*

84.   Schecter, A., Cramer, P., Boggess, K., Stanley, J., Päpke, O., Olson, J., ... Schmitz, M. (2001). Intake of Dioxins And Related Compounds From Food In The U.S. Population. *J Toxicol Environ Health A*, 63(1):1-18.

85.   Washington State University (2012). Dioxin causes disease and reproductive problems across generations, study finds. *ScienceDaily*. Retrieved from ***http://www.sciencedaily.com/releases/2012/09/120926213939.htm***

86.   Hyman, M. (2011, Feb 12). Acne: Are Milk and Sugar the Causes? Huffington Post. Retrieved from ***http://www.huffingtonpost.com/dr-mark-hyman/do-milk-and-sugar-cause-a_b_822163.html***

87.   Adebamowo, C.A., Spiegelman, D., Danby, F.W., Frazier, A.L., Willett, W.C., & Holmes, M.D. (2005). High school dietary intake and teenage acne. *J Am Acad Dermatol*, 52(2):207-214.

88.   Adebamowo, C.A., Spiegelman, D., Berkey, C.S., Danby, F.W., Rockett, H.H., Colditz, G.A., ... Holmes, M.D. (2006). Milk consumption and acne in adolescent girls. *Dermatol Online J*, 12(4):1.

89.   Lucarelli, S., Frediani, T., Zingoni, A.M., Ferruzzi, F., Giardini, O., Quintieri, F., ... Cardi, E. (1995). Food allergy and infantile autism. *Panminerva Med*, 37(3), 137-141.

90.   GFCFDiet.com. Success Stories. Retrieved from ***http://gfcfdiet.com/successstories.htm***

91.   Voskuil, D.W., Vrieling, A., van't Veer, L.J., Kampman, E., & Rookus, M.A. (2005). The insulin-like growth factor system in cancer prevention: potential of dietary intervention strategies. *Cancer Epidemiol Biomarkers Prev*, 14(1):195-203.

92.   Grant, W.B. (1998). Milk and other dietary influences on coronary heart disease. *Altern Med Rev*, 3(4):281-294.

93.   Egger, J., Carter, C.M., Wilson, J., Turner, M.W., & Soothill, J.F. (1983). Is migraine food allergy? A double-blind controlled trial of

oligoantigenic diet treatment. *Lancet*, 2(8355):865-869.

94.   Mansfield, L.E., Vaughan, T.R., Waller, S.F., Haverly, R.W., & Ting, S. (1985). Food allergy and adult migraine: double-blind and mediator confirmation of an allergic etiology. *Ann Allergy*, 55(2):126-129.

95.   Malosse, D., Perron, H., Sasco, A., & Seigneurin, J.M. (1992). Correlation between milk and dairy product consumption and multiple sclerosis prevalence: a worldwide study. *Neuroepidemiology*, 11(4-6):304-312.

96.   Malosse, D., & Perron H. (1993). Correlation analysis between bovine populations, other farm animals, house pets, and multiple sclerosis. *Neuroepidemiology*, 12(1):15-27.

97.   Faber, M.T., Jensen, A., Søgaard, M., Høgdall, E., Høgdall, C., Blaakaer, J., & Kjaer, S.K. (2012). Use of dairy products, lactose, and calcium and risk of ovarian cancer - results from a Danish case-control study. *Acta Oncol*, 51(4):454-464.

98.   Cramer, D.W., Greenberg, E.R., Titus-Ernstoff, L., Liberman, R.F., Welch, W.R., Li, E., & Ng, W.G. (2000). A case-control study of galactose consumption and metabolism in relation to ovarian cancer. *Cancer Epidemiol Biomarkers Prev*, 9(1):95-101.

99.   Genkinger, J.M., Hunter, D.J., Spiegelman, D., Anderson, K.E., Arslan, A., Beeson, W.L., … Smith-Warner, S.A. (2006). Dairy products and ovarian cancer: a pooled analysis of 12 cohort studies. *Cancer Epidemiol Biomarkers Prev*, 15(2):364-372.

100.   Chen, H., Zhang, S.M., Hernán, M.A., Willett, W.C., & Ascherio, A. (2002). Diet and Parkinson's disease: a potential role of dairy products in men. *Ann Neurol*, 52(6):793-801.

101.   Chen, H., O'Reilly, E., McCullough, M.L., Rodriguez, C., Schwatzschild, M.A., Calle, E.E., & Ascherio, A. (2007). Consumption of dairy products and risk of Parkinson's disease. *Am J Epidemiol*, 165(9):998-1006.

102.   Grant, W.B. (1999). An ecologic study of dietary links to prostate cancer. *Altern Med Rev*, 4(3):162-169.

103.   Chan, J.M., Stampfer, M.J., Ma, J., Gann, P.H., Gaziano, J.M., & Giovannucci, E.L. (2001). Dairy products, calcium, and prostate cancer risk in the Physician's Health Study. *Am J Clin Nutr*, 74(4):549-554.

104.   Davies, T.W., Palmer, C.R., Ruja, E., Lipscombe, J.M. (1996). Adolescent milk, dairy product and fruit consumption and testicular cancer. *Br J Cancer*, 74(4):657-660.

105.   Saukkonen, T., Virtanen, S.M., Karppinen, M., Reijonen, H., Ilonen, J., Räsäanen, L., ... Savilahti, E. (1998). Significance of cow's milk protein antibodies as risk factor for childhood IDDM: interactions with dietary cow's milk intake and HLA-DQB1 genotype. Childhood Diabetes in Finland Study Group. *Diabetologia*, 41(1):72-78.

106.   Kimpimäki, T., Erkkola, M., Korhonen, S., Kupila, A., Virtanen, S.M., Ilonen, J., ... Knip, M. (2001). Short-term exclusive breastfeeding predisposes young children with increased genetic risk of Type I diabetes to progressive beta-cell autoimmunity. *Diabetologia*, 44(1):63-69.

107.   Dhanwal, D.K., Dennison, E.M., Harvey, N.C., & Cooper C. (2011). Epidemiology of hip fracture: Worldwide geographic variation. *Indian J Orthop*, 45(1):15-22.

108.   Dhanwal, D.K., Cooper, C., & Dennison, E.M. (2010). Geographic variation in osteoporotic hip fracture incidence: the growing importance of asian influences in coming decades. *J Osteoporos*, 2010:757102.

109.   Barnard, Neal. (2003). *Breaking the Food Seduction: The Hidden Reasons Behind Food Cravings—-And 7 Steps to End Them Naturally*. New York, NY: St. Martin's Press.

110.   Wiley, A.S. (2011). Milk Intake and Total Dairy

Consumption: Associations with Early Menarche in NHANES 1999-2004. *PLoS ONE*, 6(2):e14685.

111.   Özen, S., & Darcan Ş. (2011). Effects of environmental endocrine disruptors on pubertal development. *J Clin Res Pediatr Endocrinol*, 3(1):1-6.

112.   Djoussé, L., Gaziano, J.M., Buring, J.E., Lee, I.M. (2009). Egg Consumption and Risk of Type 2 Diabetes in Men and Women. *Diabetes Care*, 32(2):295-300.

113.   Djoussé, L., & Gaziano, M. (2008). Egg consumption in relation to cardiovascular disease and morality: the Physician's Health Study. *Am J Clin Nutr*, 87(4):964-969.

114.   Richman, E.L., Kenfield, S.A., Stampfer, M.J., Giovannucci, E.L., & Chan J.M. (2011). Egg, red meat, poultry intake and risk of lethal prostate cancer in the prostate-specific antigen-era: incidence and survival. *Cancer Prev Res (Phila)*, 4(12):2110-2121.

115.   Zhang, J., Zhao, Z., & Berkel, H.J. (2003). Egg consumption and mortality from colon and rectal cancers: an ecological study. *Nutr Cancer*, 46(2):158-165.

116.   Steinmetz, K.A., & Potter J.D. (1994). Egg consumption and cancer of the colon and rectum. *Eur J Cancer Prev*, 3(3):237-245.

117.   Iscovich, J.M., L'Abbé, K.A., Castelleto, R., Calzona, A., Bernedo, A., Chopita, N.A., & Kaldor, J. (1992). Colon cancer in Argentina. I: Risk from intake of dietary items. *Int J Cancer*, 51(6):851-857.

118.   Radosavljević, V., Janković, S., Marinković, J., & Dokić, M. (2005). Diet and bladder cancer: a case-control study. *Int Urol Nephrol*, 37(2):283-289.

119.   Judd, N., Griffith, W.C., & Faustman, E.M. (2004). Contribution of PCB exposure from fish consumption to total dioxin-like dietary exposure. *Regul Toxicol Pharmacol*, 40(2):125-135.

120.   U.S. Public Health Service, The Agency for Toxic Substances and Disease Registry, U.S. Department of Health and Human Services, & The U.S. Environmental Protection Agency. Public Health Implications of Exposure to Polychlorinated Biphenyls (PCBs). EPA.gov. Retrieved from *http://water.epa.gov/scitech/swguidance/fishshellfish/techguidance/upload/pcb99.pdf*

121.   Scudder, B.C., Chasar, L.C., Wentz, D.A., Bauch, N.J., Bringham, M.E., Moran, P.W., ... Krabbenhoft, D.P. (2009). Mercury in Fish, Bed Sediment, and Water from Streams Across the United States, 1998-2005. U.S. Geological Survey Scientific Investigations Report 2009-5109, 74 p.

122.   Lempert, P. (2006, Dec 27). The 5 things you need to know about deli meats. TODAY.com. Retrieved from *http://today.msnbc.msn.com/id/16361276/ns/today-food/t/things-you-need-know-about-deli-meats/#.UMvb43PjmXS*

123.   Blaylock, R.L. (1997). *Excitotoxins: The Taste that Kills.* Albuquerque, NM: Health Press NA.

124.   Gallagher, D.L., Ebel, E.D., & Kause, J.R. (2003). FSIS Risk Assessment for *Listeria monocytogenes* in Deli Meats. USDA Food Safety and Inspection Service. Retrieved from *http://www.fsis.usda.gov/oppde/rdad/frpubs/97-013f/listeriareport.pdf*

125.   Rampton, R. (2008, Aug 26). Canada says 12 dead in food poisoning outbreak. *Reuters.* Retrieved from *http://www.reuters.com/article/2008/08/26/us-meat-idUSN2526525120080826?feedType=RSS&feedName=healthNews&sp=true*

126.   Barnard, N. (2001, Aug 10). Could Processed Meat Give You Cancer? HuffingtonPost.com . Retrieved from *http://www.huffingtonpost.com/neal-barnard-md/processed-meat-cancer_b_919034.html*

127.   Chan, D.S.M., Lau, R., Aune, D., Vieira, R., Greenwood, D.C., Kampman, E., & Norat, T. (2011). Red and Processed Meat and Colorectal Cancer Incidence: Meta-Analysis of Prospective Studies.

PLoS ONE, 6(6):e20456.

128.   Punnen, S., Hardin, J., Cheng, I., Klein, E.A., & Witte, J.S. (2011). Impact of Meat Consumption, Preparation, and Mutagens on Aggressive Prostate Cancer. *PLoS ONE*, 6(11):e27711.

129.   Larsson, S.C., Bergkvist, L., & Wolk, A. (2004). Milk and lactose intakes and ovarian cancer risk in the Swedish Mammography Cohort. *Am J Clin Nutr*, 80(5):1353-1357.

130.   Larsson, S.C., Orsini, N., & Wolk, A. (2006). Milk, milk products and lactose intake and ovarian cancer risk: a meta-analysis of epidemiological studies. *Int J Cancer*, 118(2):431-441.

131.   Fairfield K.M., Hunter, D.J., Colditz, G.A., Fuchs, C.S., Cramer, D.W., Speizer, F.E., ... Hankinson, S.E. (2004). A prospective study of dietary lactose and ovarian cancer. *Int J Cancer*, 110(2):271-277.

132.   Cramer, D.W., Harlow, B.L., Willett, W.C., Welch, W.R., Bell, D.A., Scully, R.E., ... Knapp, R.C. (1989). Galactose consumption and metabolism in relation to the risk of ovarian cancer. *Lancet*, 2(8654):66-71.

133.   European Lung Foundation (2011). Low-fat yogurt intake when pregnant linked to increased risk of child asthma and hay fever, study suggests. *ScienceDaily*. Retrieved from ***http://www.sciencedaily.com/releases/2011/09/110918024046.htm***

134.   WebMD (2002, April 22). High-Protein Diets Cause Dehydration. Retrieved from ***http://www.webmd.com/diet/news/20020422/high-protein-diets-cause-dehydration***

135.   Wake Forest University Baptist Medical Center (2010). Excess protein in urine is indicator of heart disease risk in whites, but not blacks, study suggests. *ScienceDaily*. Retrieved from ***http://www.sciencedaily.com/releases/2010/01/100111155104.htm***

136.   Lagiou, P., Sandin, S., Lof, M., Trichopoulos, D., Adami, H.,

& Weiderpass, E. (2012). Low carbohydrate-high protein diet and incidence of cardiovascular diseases in Swedish women: a prospective cohort study. BMJ, 344:e4026.

137.   Sellmeyer, D.E., Stone, K.L., Sebastian, A., & Cummings, S.R. (2001). A high ratio of dietary animal to vegetable protein increases the rate of bones loss and the risk of fracture in postmenopausal women. Study of Osteoporotic Fractures Research Group. *Am J Clin Nutr*, 73(1):118-122.

138.   McCarty, M.F. (1999). Vegan proteins may reduce risk of cancer, obesity, and cardiovascular disease by promoting increased glucagon activity. Med Hypotheses, 53(6):459-485.

139.   Robbins, J. (1987). *Diet for a New America: How Your Food Choices Affect Your Health, Happiness, and the Future of Life on Earth.* Tiburon, CA: H J Kramer.

140.   A Report of the Panel on Macronutrients, Subcommittees on Upper Reference Levels of Nutrients and Interpretation and Uses of Dietary Reference Intakes, Standing Committee on the Scientific Evaluation of Dietary Reference Intakes (2005). *Dietary Reference Intakes for Energy, Carbohydrate, Fiber, Fat, Fatty Acids, Cholesterol, Protein, and Amino Acids (Macronutrients).* Washington, DC: The National Academies Press.

141.   Bender, A. (1998). Meat and meat products in human nutrition in developing countries. Food and Agriculture Organization of the United Nations. Retrieved from ***http://www.fao.org/docrep/ t0562e/T0562E00.htm#Contents***

142.   Greger, M. (2012, Jul 24). The Benefit of Calorie Restricting Without the Actual Restricting. NutritionFacts.org. Retrieved from ***http://nutritionfacts.org/video/the-benefits-of-caloric-restriction- without-the-actual-restricting/***

143.   Held, L.E. (2012, March 1). Do vegans burn more calories? Retrieved from ***http://www.wellandgoodnyc.com/2012/03/01/do- vegans-burn-more-calories/#***

144.   Barnard, N.D., Cohen, J., Jenkins, D.J.A., Turner-McGrievy, G., Gloede, L., Jaster, B., ... Talpers, S. (2006). A Low-Fat Vegan Diet Improves Glycemic Control and Cardiovascular Risk Factors in a Randomized Clinical Trial in Individuals With Type 2 Diabetes. Diabetes Care, 29(8):1777-1783.

145.   Hänninen, O., Kaartinen, K., Rauma, A.L., Nenonen, M., Törrönen, Häkkinen, S., ... Laakso, J. (2000). Antioxidants in vegan diet and rheumatic disorders. *Toxicology*, 155(1-3):45-53.

146.   Tantamango-Bartley, Y., Jaceldo-Siegl, K., Fan, J., & Fraser, G. (2012). Vegetarian Diets and the Incidence of Cancer in a Low-Risk Population. *Cancer Epidemiol Biomarkers Prev.* [Epub ahead of print]

147.   The University of Chicago (2006, April 13). Study: vegan diets healthier for planet, people than meat diets. Retrieved from ***http://www-news.uchicago.edu/releases/06/060413.diet.shtml***

148.   Fiala, N. (2009, Feb 4). How Meat Contributes to Global Warming. Scientific American. Retrieved from ***http://www.scientificamerican.com/slideshow.cfm?id=the-greenhouse-hamburger#3***

149.   Thomassen, M.A., van Calker, K.J., Smits, M.C.J., Iepema, G.L., & de Boer, I.J.M. (2008). Life cycle assessment of conventional and organic milk production in the Netherlands. Agricultural Systems, 96(1-3):95-107.

150.   Raloff, J. (2009, Feb 15). AAAS: Climate-friendly dining ... meats: The carbon footprints of raising livestock for food. *ScienceNews*. Retrieved from ***http://www.sciencenews.org/view/generic/id/40934/title/AAAS_Climate-friendly_dining_%E2%80%A6_meats***

151.   Cui, S., Ge, B., Zheng, J., & Meng, J. (2005). Prevalence and Antimicrobial Resistance of *Campylobacter* spp. and *Salmonella* Serovars in Organic Chickens from Maryland Retail Stores. *Appl Environ Microbiol*, 71(7):4108-4111.

152.   Joy, M. (2010). *Why We Love Dogs, Eat Pigs and Wear Cows: An Introduction to Carnism*. San Francisco, CA: Conari Press

153.   American Association For The Advancement Of Science (2001). Diet And Disease In Cattle: High-Grain Feed May Promote Illness And Harmful Bacteria. *ScienceDaily*. Retrieved from ***http://www.sciencedaily.com/releases/2001/05/010511074623.htm***

154.   Roberts, J.L. (1982). The prevalence and economic significance of liver disorders and contamination in grain-fed and grass-fed cattle. *Aust Vet J*, 59(5):129-132.

155.   People for the Ethical Treatment of Animals. The Beef Industry. Retrieved from ***http://www.peta.org/issues/animals-used-for-food/beef-industry.aspx***

156.   The American Society for the Prevention of Cruelty to Animals. Farm Animal Cruelty Glossary. Retrieved from ***http://www.aspca.org/fight-animal-cruelty/farm-animal-cruelty/farm-animal-cruelty-glossary.aspx#debeaking***

157.   United Poultry Concerns. Debeaking. Retrieved from ***http://www.upc-online.org/merchandise/debeak_factsheet.html***

158.   People for the Ethical Treatment of Animals. Commercial Fishing: How Fish Get From the High Seas to Your Supermarket. Retrieved from ***http://www.peta.org/issues/animals-used-for-food/commercial-fishing.aspx***

159.   Greger, M. (2012, Jul 26). Uprooting the Leading Causes of Death. Retrieved from ***http://www.youtube.com/watch?v=30gEiweaAVQ***

Chapter 2: Why Low-Fat?

1.   People for the Ethical Treatment of Animals. Accidentally Vegan. Retrieved from ***http://www.peta.org/living/vegetarian-living/Accidentally-Vegan.aspx***

2.   Adams, M. (2004, Jul 24). Many "healthy" and vegetarian foods contain MSG in the form of yeast extract. NaturalNews. Retrieved from ***http://www.naturalnews.com/001528.html***

3.   Care2.com Contributor. 10 Surprising Sources of MSG. Retrieved from ***http://recipes.howstuffworks.com/10-surprising-sources-of-msg.htm***

4.   Willet, W.C. (2012). Dietary fats and coronary heart disease. *J Intern Med*, 272(1):13-24.

5.   Oh, K, Hu, F.B., Manso, J.E., Stampfer, M.J., & Willett, W.C. (2005). Dietary Fat Intake and Risk of Coronary Heart Disease in Women: 20 Years of Follow-Up of the Nurses' Health Study. *Am J Epidemiol*, 161(7):672-679.

6.   Sun, Q., Ma, J., Campos, H., Hankinson, S.E., Manson, J.E., Stampfer, M.J., ... Hu, F.B. (2007). A Prospective Study of Trans Fatty Acids in Erythrocytes and Risk of Coronary Heart Disease. *Circulation*, 115:1858-1865.

7.   Imamura, F., Lemaitre, R.N., King, I.B., Song, X., Lichtenstein, A.H., Matthan, N.R., ... Mozaffarian, D. (2012). Novel circulating fatty acid patterns and risk of cardiovascular disease: the Cardiovascular Health Study. *Am J Clin Nutr*, 96(6):1252-1261.

8.   Willett, W.C., & Mozaffarian, D. (2007). Trans fat in cardiac and diabetes risk: an overview. *Current Cardiovascular Risk Reports*, 1(1):16-23.

9.   Odegaard, A.O., & Pereira, M.A. (2006). Trans fatty acids, insulin resistance, and type 2 diabetes. *Nutr Rev*, 64(8):364-372.

10.   Salmerón, J, Hu, F.B., Stampfer, M.J., Colditz, G.A., Rimm, E.B., & Willett, W.C. (2001). Dietary fat intake and risk of type 2 diabetes in women. *Am J Clin Nutr*, 73(6):1019-1026.

11.   Kavanagh, K., Jones, K.L., Sawyer, J., Kelley, K., Carr, J.J., Wagner, J.D., & Rudel, L.L. (2007). Trans Fat Diet Induces Abdominal Obesity and Changes in Insulin Sensitivity in Monkeys. *Obesity*, 15:1675-1684.

12.   Hu, J., La Vecchia, C., de Groh, M., Negri, E., Morrison, H.,

Mery, L., & Canadian Cancer Registries Epidemiology Research Group (2011). Dietary transfatty acids and cancer risk. *Eur J Cancer Prev*, 20(6):530-538.

13.   Gilsing, A.M.J., Weijenberg, M.P., Goldbohm, R.A., van den Brandt, P., & Schouten, L.J. (2011). Consumption of dietary fat and meat and risk of ovarian cancer in the Netherlands Cohort Study. *Am J Clin Nutr*, 93(1), 118-126.

14.   Hu, J., La Vecchia, C., Gibbons, L., Negri, E., Mery, L. (2010). Nutrients and risk of prostate cancer. *Nutr Cancer*, 62(6):710-718.

15.   Morris, M.C., Evans, D.A., Bienias, J.L., Tangney, C.C., Bennett, D.A., Aggarwal, N., ... Wilson, R.S. (2003). Dietary fats and the risk of incident Alzheimer disease. *Arch Neurol*, 60(2):194-200.

16.   Sánchez-Villega, A., Verberne, L., De Irala, J., Ruíz-Canela, M., Toledo, E., Serra-Marjem, L. & Martínez-González, M.A. (2011). Dietary Fat Intake and the Risk of Depression: The SUN Project. *PLoS ONE*, 6(1):e16268.

17.   Golomb, B.A., Evans, M.A., White, H.L., & Dimsdale, J.E. (2012). Trans fat consumption and aggression. *PLoS ONE*, 7(3):e32175.

18.   Physicians Committee for Responsible Medicine. Permanent Weight Control. Retrieved from ***http://www.pcrm.org/health/health-topics/permanent-weight-control***

19.   Fuhrman, J. Nutrient Density. Retrieved from ***http://www.drfuhrman.com/library/article17.aspx***

20.   Simopoulos, A.P. (2002). The importance of the ratio of omega-6/omega-3 essential fatty acids. *Biomed Pharmacother*, 56(8):365-379.

21.   Simopoulos, A.P. (2008). The Importance of the Omega-6/Omega-3 Fatty Acid Ratio in Cardiovascular Disease and Other Chronic Diseases. *Exp Biol Med*, 233(6):674-688.

22.   Norris, J. (2012). Omega-3 Fatty Acid Recommendations for Vegetarians. VeganHealth.org. Retrieved from *http://www. veganhealth.org/articles/omega3*

23.   Fuhrman, J. Dr. Fuhrman's DHA+EPA Purity. Retrieved from *http://www.drfuhrman.com/shop/DHA_EPA.aspx*

24.   American Society for BIochemistry and Molecular Biology (2009). Omega Fatty Acid Balance Can Alter Immunity And Gene Expression. *ScienceDaily*. Retrieved from *http://www.sciencedaily. com/releases/2009/05/090529183250.htm*

25.   Simopoulos, A.P. (2002). Omega-3 Fatty Acids in Inflammation and Autoimmune Diseases. *J Am Coll Nutr*, 21(6):495-505.

26.   Ramsden, C.E., Hibbeln, J.R., Majchrzak, S.F., & Davis, J.M. (2010). n-6 fatty acid-specific and mixed polyunsaturate dietary interventions have different effects on CHD risk: a meta-analysis of randomised controlled trials. *Br J Nutr*, 104(11):1586-1600.

27.   CNRS (2010). Excessive intake of omega 6 and deficiencies in omega 3 induce obesity down the generations. *ScienceDaily*. Retrieved from *http://www.sciencedaily.com/releases/2010/07/100726221737. htm*

28.   Patterson, E., Wall, R., Fitzgerald, G.F., Ross, R.P., & Stanton, C. (2012). Health implications of high dietary omega-6 polyunsaturated Fatty acids. *J Nutr Metab*, 2012:539426.

29.   de Batlle, J., Sauleda, J., Balcells, E., Gómez, F.P., Méndez, M., Rodriguez, E., ... PAC-COPD Study Group. (2012). Association between Ω3 and Ω6 fatty acid intakes and serum inflammatory markers in COPD. *J Nutr Biochem*, 23(7):817-821.

30.   Sonestedt, E., Ericson, U., Gullberg, B., Skog, K., Olsson, H., & Wirfält, E. (2008). Do both heterocyclic amines and omega-6 polyunsaturated fatty acids contribute to the incidence of breast cancer in postmenopausal women of the Malmö diet and cancer

cohort. *Int J Cancer*, 123(7):1637-1643.

31.   University of California (2005). Omega-6 Fatty Acids Cause Prostate Tumor Cell Growth in Culture. *ScienceDaily*. Retrieved from *http://www.sciencedaily.com/releases/2005/08/050802123505.htm*

32.   Kris-Etherton, P.M., Taylor, D.S., Yu-Poth, S., Huth, P., Moriarty, K., Fishell, V., … Etherton, T,D. (2000). Polyunsaturated fatty acids in the food chain in the United States. *Am J Clin Nutr*, 71(1 Suppl): 179S-1788S.

33.   Norris, J. (2010, Nov 8). DHA Supplements: A Good Idea, Especially for Older Vegan Men. Retrieved from *http://jacknorrisrd.com/?p=1553*

34.   Sabaté, J., Oda, K., & Ros., E. (2010). Nut consumption and blood lipid levels: a pooled analysis of 25 intervention trials. *Arch Intern Med*, 170(9):821-827.

35.   McDougall, J. McDougall Program Success Stories. Retrieved from *http://www.drmcdougall.com/stars/index.html*

36.   Fuhrman, J. Success Stories. Retrieved from *http://www.drfuhrman.com/success/stories.aspx/7?query=cholesterol*

37.   *Encyclopædia* Britannica (2012) insulin. Retrieved from *http://www.britannica.com/EBchecked/topic/289486/insulin*

38.   National Diabetes Information Clearinghouse (2011). Insulin Resistance and Prediabetes. Retrieved from *http://diabetes.niddk.nih.gov/dm/pubs/insulinresistance/*

39.   Van Beek, M., Oravecz-Wilson, K.I., Delekta, P.C., Gu, S., Li, X., Jin, X., … Lucas, P.C. (2012). Bcl10 links saturated fat overnutrition with hepatocellular NF-kB activation and insulin resistance. *Cell Rep*, 1(5):444-452.

40.   Mayer, E.J., Newman, B., Quesenberry, C.P. Jr., & Selby, J.V. (1993). Usual dietary fat intake and insulin concentrations in healthy women twins. *Diabetes Care*, 16(11):1459-1469.

41.   Rahman, K. (2007). Studies on free radicals, antioxidants, and co-factors. *Clin Interv Aging*, 2(2):219-236.

42.   Blankenhorn, D.H., Johnson, R.L., Mack, W.J., el Zein, H.A., & Vailas, L.I. (1990). The influences of diet on the appearance of new lesions in human coronary arteries. *JAMA*, 263(12):1646-1652.

43.   Larsen, L.F., Bladbjerg, E.M., Jespersen, J., & Marckman, P. (1997). Effects of Dietary Fat Quality and Quantity on Postprandial Activation of Blood Coagulation Factor VII. *Arterioscler Thromb Vasc Biol*, 17(11):2904-2909.

44.   Esselstyn, Caldwell B. Jr. (2007). *Prevent and Reverse Heart Disease: The Revolutionary, Scientifically Proven, Nutrition-Based Cure.* New York, NY: Penguin Group.

45.   McDougall, J.A., & McDougall, M. (2012). The Starch Solution: Eat the Foods You Love, Regain Your Health, and Lose the Weight for Good! New York, NY: Rodale Books.

46.   Barnard, Neal. (2003). *Breaking the Food Seduction: The Hidden Reasons Behind Food Cravings—-And 7 Steps to End Them Naturally.* New York, NY: St. Martin's Press.

47.   Ornish, D. (2007). The Spectrum: A Scientifically Proven Program to Feel Better, Live Longer, Lose Weight, and Gain Health. New York, NY: Ballantine Books.

48.   Graham, D.N. (2006). The 80/10/10 Diet: Balancing Your Health, Your Weight, and Your Life, One Luscious Bite at a Time. Key Largo, FL: FoodnSport Press

49.   Physicians Committee for Responsible Medicine. Frequently Asked Questions About Diabetes. Retrieved from ***http://www.pcrm.org/health/diabetes-resources/frequently-asked-questions-about-diabetes***

50.   Campbell, C.T. Fat and Plant-Based Diets. Retrieved from ***http://www.tcolincampbell.org/courses-resources/article/fat-and-***

plant-based-diets/?tx_ttnews%5BbackPid%5D=76&cHash=0572c53e9
7cbb87835c491716c1cb9e0

51.   Fuhrman, J. Dr. Fuhrman's Nutritarian Pyramid. Retrieved from *http://www.drfuhrman.com/library/foodpyramid.aspx#.*
UM1ZYnPjmXR

52.   Bramen, L. (2010, Feb 10). The Evolution of the Sweet Tooth. Smithsonian.com. Retrieved from *http://blogs.smithsonianmag.com/*
food/2010/02/the-evolution-of-the-sweet-tooth/

53.   Holt, S.H., Delargy, H.J., Lawton, C.L., & Blundell, J.E. (1999). The effects of high-carbohydrate vs high-fat breakfast on feelings of fullness and alertness, and subsequent food intake. *Int J Food Sci Nutr*, 50(1):13-28.

54.   Cotton, J.R., Burley, V.J., Weststrate, J.A., & Blundell, J.E. (2007). Dietary fat and appetite: similarities and differences in the satiating effect of meals supplemented with either fat or carbohydrate. *J Hum Nutr Diet*, 20(3):186-199.

55.   Flint, A., Raben, A., Astrup, A., & Holst, J.J. (1998). Glucagon-like peptide 1 promotes satiety and suppressed energy intake in humans. *J Clin Invest*, 101(3):515-520.

56.   Lavin, J.H., & Read, N.W. (1995). The effect of hunger and satiety of slowing the absorption of glucose: relationship with gastric emptying and postprandial blood glucose and insulin responses. *Appetite*, 25(1):89-96.

Chapter 3: Why Raw?

1.   Pickrell, J. (2005, Feb 19). Human 'dental chaos' linked to evolution of cooking. *NewScientist*. Retrieved from *http://www.*
newscientist.com/article/dn7035

2.   Larsen, C.P. (2002). Post-Pleistocene Human Evolution: Bioarcheology of the Agricultural Transition. In P.S. Ungar, & M.F. Teaford (Eds.), *Human Diet: It's origin and Evolution* (pp. 19-35). Westport, CT: Bergin and Garvey.

3.   Lucas, P.W. (2007) The Evolution of the Hominin Diet from a Dental Functional Perspective. In P.S. Ungar (Ed), *Evolution of the Human Diet* (pp. 31-38). New York, NY: Oxford University Press.

4.   Walker, A. (2007) Early Hominin Diets: Overview and Historical Perspectives. In P.S. Ungar (Ed), *Evolution of the Human Diet* (pp. 31-38). New York, NY: Oxford University Press.

5.   Perry, G.H., Dominy, N.J., Claw, K.G., Lee, A.S., Fiegler, H., Redon, R., ... Stone, A.C. (2007). Diet and evolution of human amylase gene copy number variation. *Nat Genet*, 39(10):1256-1260.

6.   O'Connell, J., Hawkes, K., & Jones, N.B. (2002). Meat-Eating, Grandmothering, and the Evolution of Early Human Diets. In P.S. Ungar, & M.F. Teaford (Eds.), *Human Diet: It's origin and Evolution* (pp. 19-35). Westport, CT: Bergin and Garvey.

7.   Wrangham, R. (2009). *Catching Fire: How Cooking Made Us Human*. New York, NY: Basic Books.

8.   Wolfe, D. (2012). *The Sunfood Diet Success System* (9th ed.). Berkeley, CA: NorthAtlantic Books.

9.   Clement, B.R. & DiGeronimo, T.F. (1998). *Living Foods for Optimum Health: Your Complete Guide to the Healing Power of Raw Foods*. New York, NY: Three Rivers Press.

10.   Howell, E. (1985). Enzyme Nutrition: The Food Enzyme Concept. USA: Howell, Edward.

11.   Steenkamp, G., & Gorrel, C. (1999). Oral and dental conditions in adult African wild dog skulls: a preliminary report. *J Vet Dent*, 16(2):65-68.

12.   Greer, M., Greer, J.K., & Gillingham, J. (1977). Osteoarthritis in Selected Wild Animals. Proceedings of the Oklahoma Academy of Science, 57:39-43.

13.   Hampl, J.S., Taylor, C.A., & Johnstone, C.S. (2004). Vitamin C Deficiency and Depletion in the United States: The Third National

Health and Nutrition Examination Survey, 1988 to 1994. *Am J Public Health*, 94(5):870-875.

14.   Forrest, K.Y., & Stuhldreher, W.L. (2011). Prevalence and correlates of vitamin D deficiency in US adults. *Nutr Res*, 31(1):48-54.

15.   Tufts University, Health Sciences (2008). Trends of Vitamin B6 Status in the US Population Sample Identified. *ScienceDaily*. Retrieved from ***http://www.sciencedaily.com/releases/2008/05/080520103435.htm***

16.   Allen, L.H. (2009). How common is vitamin B-12 deficiency? *Am J Clin Nutr*, 89(2): 693S-696S.

17.   Centers for Disease Control and Prevention (2011, Feb 23). Iron and Iron Deficiency. Retrieved from ***http://www.cdc.gov/nutrition/everyone/basics/vitamins/iron.html***

18.   MedlinePlus (2012, Aug 1). Rickets. Retrieved from ***http://www.nlm.nih.gov/medlineplus/ency/article/000344.htm***

19.   Norris, J. Overt B12 Deficiency - Nerve Damage and Anemia. Retrieved from ***http://www.veganhealth.org/b12/sympt***

20.   Davis, B., & Melina, V. (2010). *Becoming Raw: The Essential Guide to Raw Vegan Diets*. Summertown, TN: Book Publishing Company.

21.   Shortle, D. (1996). The denatured state (the other half of the folding equation) and its role in protein stability. *The FASEB Journal*, 10(1):27-34.

22.   Rehman, Z., & Shah, W.H. (2005). Thermal heat processing effects on antinutrients, protein and starch digestibility of food legumes. *Food Chemistry*, 91(2): 327-331.

23.   Kouchakoff, P. (1930). The Influence of Food Cooking on the Blood Formula of Man. First International Congress of Microbiology, Paris.

24.   Galgano, F., Favati, F., Caruso, M., Pietrafesa, A., & Natella, S. (2007). The influence of processing and preservation on the retention of health-promoting compounds in broccoli. *J Food Sci*, 72(2):S130-S135.

25.   Pellegrini, N., Chiavaro, E., Gardana, C., Mazzeo, T., Contino, D., … Porrini, M. (2010). Effect of different cokking methods on color, phytochemical concentration, and antioxidant capacity of raw and frozen brassica vegetables. *J Agric Food Chem*, 58(7):4310-4321.

26.   Tarwadi, K., & Agte, V. (2003). Potential of commonly consumed green leafy vegetables for their antioxidant capacity and its linkage with the micronutrient profile. *Int J Food Sci Nutr*, 54(6);417-425.

27.   Porter, Y. (2012). Antioxidant properties of green broccoli and purple-sprouting broccoli under different cooking conditions. *Bioscience Horizons*, 5:hzs004.

28.   McKillop, D.J., Pentieva, K., Daly, D., McPartlin, J.M., Hughes, J., Strain, J.J., … McNulty, H. (2002). The effect of different cooking methods on folate retention in various foods that are amongst the major contributors to folate intake in the UK diet. *Br J Nutr*, 88(6):681-688.

29.   Rock, C.L., Lovalvo, J.L., Emenhiser, C., Ruffin, M.T., Flatt, S.W., & Schwartz, S.J. (1998). Bioavailability of beta-carotene is lower in raw than in processed carrots and spinach in women. *J Nutr*, 128(5):913-916.

30.   Link, L.B., & Potter, J.D. (2004). Raw versus cooked vegetables and cancer risk. *Cancer Epidemiol Biomarkers Prev*, 13(9):1422-1435.

31.   O'Brien, J., & Morrissey, P.A. (1989). Nutritional and toxicological aspects of the Maillard browning reaction in foods. *Crit Rev Food Sci Nutr*, 28(3):211-248.

32.   Słupski, J. (2010). Effect of cooking and sterilisation on the

composition of amino acids in immature seeds of flageolet bean (Phaseolus vulgaris L.) cultivars. *Food Chemistry*, 121(4).

33.   Van Barneveld, R.J., Batterham, E.S., & Norton, B.W. (1994). The effect of heat on amino acids for growing pigs. 3. The availability of lysine from heat-treated field peas (Pisum sativum cultivar Dundale) determined using the slope-ratio assay. *Br J Nutr*, 72(2):257-275.

34.   Clemente, A., Sánchez-Vioque, R., Vioque, J., Bautista, J., & Millán, F. (1998). Effect of cooking on protein quality of chickpea (*Cicer arietinum*) seeds. *Food Chemistry*, 62(1):1-6.

35.   Zhang, J.J., Ji, R., Hu, Y.Q., Chen, J.C., & Ye, X.Q. (2011). Effect of three cooking methods on nutrient components and antioxidant capacities of bamboo shoot (Phyllostachys praecox C.D. Chu et C.S. Chao). *J Zhejiang Univ Sci B*, 12(9):752-759.

36.   Foster, S. (2011). Is Apple Cider Vinegar Healthy? Retrieved from ***http://www.fitonraw.com/2011/03/apple-cider-vinegar-is-not-a-health-food/***

37.   Khanum, F., Siddalinga, S.M., Sudarshana Krishna, K.R., Santhanam, K., & Viswanathan, K.R. (2000). Dietary fiber contant of commonly fresh and cooked vegetables consumed in India. *Plant Foods Hum Nutr*, 55(3):207-218.

38.   Moore, M.A., Park, C.B., & Tsuda, H. (1998). Soluble and insoluble fiber influences on cancer development. *Crit Rev Oncol Hematol*, 27(3):229-242.

39.   Harris, P.J., Roberton, A.M., Watson, M.E., Triggs, C.M., & Ferguson, L.R. (1993). The effects of soluble-fiber polysaccharides on the adsorption of hydrophobic carcinogen to an insoluble dietary fiber. *Nutr Cancer*, 19(1):43-54.

40.   Phillips, D.H. (1999). Polycyclic aromatic hydrocarbons in the diet. *Mutat Res*, 443(1-2):139-147.

41.	Paraíba, L.C., Queiroz, S.C., Maia Ade, H., & Ferracini, V.L. (2010). Bioconcentration factor estimates of polycyclic aromatic hydrocarbons in grains of corn plant cultivated in soils treated with sewage sludge. *Sci Total Environ*, 408(16):3270-3276.

42.	Chuyen, N.V. (2006). Toxicity of the AGEs generated from the Maillard reaction: on the relationship of food-AGEs biological-AGEs. *Mol Nutr Food Res*, 50(12):1140-1149.

43.	Lineback, D.R., Coughlin, J.R., & Stadler, R.H. (2012). Acrylamide in foods: a review of the science and future considerations. *Annu Rev Food Sci Technol*, 3:15-35.

44.	Food and Agriculture Organization of the United Nations & World Health Organization (2005). Jont FAO/WHO Expert Committee on Food Additives. Retrieved from ***http://www.who.int/foodsafety/chem/jecfa/summaries/summary_report_64_final.pdf***

45.	World Health Organization. Frequently asked questions - acrylamide in food. Retrieved from ***http://www.who.int/foodsafety/publications/chem/acrylamide_faqs/en/index.html***

46.	National Cancer Institute. Acrylamide in Food and Cancer Risk. Retrieved from ***http://www.cancer.gov/cancertopics/factsheet/Risk/acrylamide-in-food#ques7***

47.	Petersen, B. (2003). Acrylamide: Formation, Exposure, Possible Reduction Strategies. Food and Agriculture Organization of the United Nations. Retrieved from ***http://www.fao.org/ag/agn/jecfa/acrylamide/petersen/tsld001.htm***

48.	Tateo, F., Bononi, M., & Andreoli, G. (2007). Acrylamide levels in cooked rice, tomato sauces, and some fast food on the Italian market. *Journal Food Composition and Analysis*, 20(3-4):232-235.

49.	Yaacoub, R., Saliba, R., Nsouli, B., Khalaf, G., & Birlouez-Aragon, I. (2008). Formation of lipid oxidation and isomerization products during processing of nuts and sesame seeds. *J Agric Food Chem*, 56(16):7082-7090.

50.   Eng, M. (2012, Mar 7). Has your food gone rancid? Consumers may have kitchen full of dangerous products and not know it. ChicagoTribune.com. Retrieved from ***http:// articles.chicagotribune.com/2012-03-07/features/sc-food-0302-rancidity-20120307_1_trans-fats-polyunsaturated-oils-food-chain***

51.   Friedman, M. (2003). Chemistry, Biochemistry, and Safety of Acrylamide. A Review. *J Agric Food Chem*, 51(16):4504-4526.

52.   Peppa, M., & Raptis, S.A. (2008). Advanced glycation end products and cardiovascular disease. *Curr Diabetes Rev*, 4(2), 92-100.

53.   Sasaki, N., Fukatsu, R., Tsuzuki, K., Hayashi, Y., Yoshida, T., Fujii, N., ... Makita, Z. (1998). Advanced glycation end products in Alzheimer's disease and other neurodegenerative diseases. *Am J Pathol*, 153(4):1149-1455.

54.   Mayo Clinic staff (2011, Jan 7). Dehydration. MayoClinic. com. Retrieved from ***http://www.mayoclinic.com/health/dehydration/ DS00561/DSECTION=symptoms***

55.   Tierney, J. (2011, Aug 17). Do You Suffer From Decision Fatigue? NYTimes.com. Retrieved from ***http://www.nytimes. com/2011/08/21/magazine/do-you-suffer-from-decision-fatigue. html?_r=5&pagewanted=1&***

56.   Campbell, C. T., & Campbell, T. M. (2006). *The China Study: Starling Implications for Diet, Weight Loss and Long-Term Health.* Dallas, TX: BenBella Books.

57.   Ferriss, T. (2010). The 4-Hour Body: An Uncommon Guide to Rapid Fat-Loss, Incredible Sex, and Becoming Superhuman [Audiobook]. Random House Audio.

58.   Wijers, S.L.J., Schrauwen, P., Saris, W.H.M., & van Marken Lichtenbelt, W.D. (2008). Human Skeletal Muscle Mitochondrial Uncoupling Is Associated with Cold Induced Adaptive Thermogenesis. *PLoS ONE*, 3(3):e1777.

59.   Fuhrman, J. (2003). *Eat To Live: The Revolutionary Formula for Fast and Sustained Weight Loss.* New York, NY: Little, Brown and Company.

60.   Block, G., Patterson, B., & Subar A. (1992). Fruit, vegetables, and cancer prevention: a review of the epidemiological evidence. *Nutr Cancer*, 18(1):1-29.

61.   Heber, D. (2004). Vegetables, fruits, and phytoestrogens in the prevention of diseases. *Journal of Postgraduate Medicine*, 50(2):145-149.

62.   Lee J.E., Männistö, S., Spiegelman, D., Hunter, D.J., Bernstein, L., can den Brandt, P.A., ... Smith-Warner, S.A. (2009). Intakes of fruit, vegetables, and carotenoids and renal cell cancer risk: a pooled analysis of 13 prospective studies. *Cancer Epidemiol Biomarkers Prev*, 18(6):1730-1739.

63.   Higdon, J. (2005). Fruits and Vegetables. Linus Pauling Institute. Retrieved from ***http://lpi.oregonstate.edu/infocenter/foods/fruitveg/#cvd***

64.   He, K., Hu, F.B., Colditz, G.A., Manson, J.E., Willett, W.C., & Lie, S. (2004). *Int J Obes Relat Disord*, 28(12):1569-1574.

65.   Vioque, J., Weinbrenner, T., Castelló, A, Asensio, L., Garcia de la Hera, M. (2008). Intake of fruits and vegetables in relation to 10-year weight gain among Spanish adults. *Obesity (Silver Spring)*, 16(3):664-670.

66.   Alinia S., Hels, O., & Tetens, I. (2009). The potential association between fruit intake and body weight—a review. *Obes Rev*, 10(6):639-647.

67.   Boffetta, P., Couto, E., Wichmann, J., Ferrari, P., Trichopoulos, D., Bueno-de-Mesquita, H.B., ... Trichopoulou, A. (2010). Fruit and vegetable intake and overall cancer risk in the European Prospective Investigation into Cancer and Nutrition (EPIC). *J Natl cancer Inst*, 102(8):529-537.

68.   Dawson-Hughes, B., Harris, S.S., & Ceglia, L. (2008). Alkaline diets favor lean tissue mass in older adults. *Am J Clin Nutr*, 87(3):662-665.

69.   Wiederkehr, M., & Krapf R. (2001). Metabolic and endocrine effects of metabolic acidosis in humans. *Swiss Med Wkly*, 131(9-10):127-132.

70.   Frassetto, L.A., Todd, K.M., Morris, R.C. Jr., & Sebastian, A. (2000). Worldwide incidence of hip fracture in elderly women: relation to consumption of animal and vegetable foods. *J Gerontol A Biol Sci Med Sci*, 55(10):M585-M592.

71.   Rensselaer Polytechnic Institute (RPI) (2012). Battling brittle bones with ... broccoli and spinach?. *ScienceDaily*. Retrieved from *http://www.sciencedaily.com/releases/2012/12/121211130210.htm*

72.   Food and Agriculture Organization of the United Nations (2006). Livestock impacts on the environment. Retrieved from *http://www.fao.org/ag/magazine/0612sp1.htm*

Chapter 4: All Raw Foods Are Not Equal

1.   Davis, B., & Melina, V. (2010). *Becoming Raw: The Essential Guide to Raw Vegan Diets*. Summertown, TN: Book Publishing Company.

2.   Weil, A. (2012, Oct 1). Q & A Library: Is Carrageenan Safe? Retrieved from *http://www.drweil.com/drw/u/QAA401181/Is-Carrageenan-Safe.html*

3.   Rukma Reddy, N.R., Sathe, S.K. (2002). *Food Phytates*. Boca Raton, FL: CRC Press

4.   Macfarlane, B.J., Bezwoda, W.R., Bothwell, T.H., Baynes, R.D., Bothwell, J.E., MacPhail, A.P., ... Mayet, F. (1988). Inhibitory effect of nuts on iron absorption. *Am J Clin Nutr*, 47(2):270-274.

5.   Weaver, C.M., Heaney, R.P., Martin, B.R., & Fitzsimmons, M.L. (1991). Human calcium absorption from whole-wheat products.

J Nutr, 121(11):1769-1775.

6.   Hallberg, L., Brune, M., & Rossander, L. (1989). Iron absorption in man: ascorbic acid and dose-dependent inhibition by phytate. *Am J Clin Nutr*, 49(1):140-144.

7.   Bohn, T., Davidsson, L., Walczyk, T., & Hurrell, R.F. (2004). Phytic acid added to white-wheat bread inhibits fractional apparent magnesium absorption in humans. Am J Clin Nutr, 79(3):418-423.

8.   Davidsson, L., Almgren, A., Juillerat, M.A., & Hurrell, R.F. (1995). Manganese absorption in humans: the effect of phytic acid ascorbic acid in soy formula. *Am J Clin Nutr*, 62(5):984-987.

9.   Adams, C.L., Hambridge, M., Raboy, V., Dorsch, J.A., Sian, L., Westcott, J.L., & Krebs, N.F. (2002). Zinc absorption from a low-phytic acid maize. *Am J Clin Nutr*, 76(3):556-559.

10.   World Health Organization (2008). Worldwide Prevalence of Anaemia 1993-2005: WHO Global Database on Anaemia. Retrieved from ***http://whqlibdoc.who.int/publications/2008/9789241596657_eng.pdf***

11.   Sharma, A., & Khetarpaul, N. (1995). Fermentation of rice-bengal gram dhal blends with whey: changes in phytic acid content and in vitro digestibility of starch protein. *Nahrung*, 39(4):282-287.

12.   Gilani, G.S., Cockell, K.A., & Sepehr, E. (2005). Effects of antinutritional factors on protein digestibility and amino acid availability in foods. *A AOAC Int*, 88(3):967-987.

13.   Kumar, V., Sinha, A.K., Makkar, H.P.S., & Becker, K. (2010). Dietary roles of phytate and phytase in human nutrition: A review. *Food Chemistry*, 120(4):945-959.

14.   Fälth-Magnusson, K., & Magnusson, K.E. (1995). Elevated levels of serum antibodies to the lectin wheat germ agglutinin in celiac children lend support to the gluten-lectin theory of celiac disease. *Pediatr Allergy Immunol*, 6(2):98-102.

15.   Ramadass, B., Dokladny, K., Moseley, P.L., Patel, Y.R., & Lin, H.C. (2010). Sucrose co-administration reduces the toxic effect of lectin on gut permeability and intestinal bacterial colonization. *Dig Dis Sci*, 55(10):2778-2784.

16.   Hamid, R., & Masood, A. (2009). Dietary Lectins as Disease Causing Toxicants. *Pakistan Journal of Nutrition*, 8(3):293-303.

17.   Freed, D.L.J. (1999). Do dietary lectins cause disease? *BMJ*, 318(7190):1023-1024.

18.   Cordain, L., Toohey, L., Smith, M.J., & Hickey, M.S. (2000). Modulation of immune function by dietary lectins in rheumatoid arthritis. *British Journal of Nutrition*, 83(3):207-217.

19.   Jönsson, T., Olsson, S., Ahrén, B., Bøg-Hansen, T., Dole, A., & Lindeberg, S. (2005). Agrarian diet and disease of affluence - Do evolutionary novel dietary lectins cause leptin resistance? *BMC Endocrine Disorders*, 5:10.

20.   Lydiard, R.B. (2001). Irritable bowel syndrome, anxiety, and depression: what are the links? *J Clin Psychiatry*, 62 Suppl 8:38-45.

21.   Dykes, L., & Rooney, L.W. (2007). Phenolic Compounds in Cereal Grains and Their Health Benefits. *Cereal Foods World*, 52(3).

22.   Afify, Ael-M, El-Beltagi, H.S., El-Salam, S.M., & Omran, A.A. (2011). Bioavailability of iron, zinc, phytate and phytase activity during soaking and germination of white sorghum varieties. *PLoS ONE*, 6(10):e25512.

23.   Haard, N.F., Odunfa, S.A., & Lee, C. (1999). Fermented Cereals. A Global Perspective. Food and Agriculture Organization of the United Nations. Retrieved from ***http://www.fao.org/docrep/x2184e/x2184e00.htm#con***

24.   PubMed Health (2012, Jan 20). Celiac disease - sprue. Retrieved from ***http://www.ncbi.nlm.nih.gov/pubmedhealth/PMH0001280/***

25.   Biesiekierski, J.R., Newnham, E.D., Irving, P.M., Barrett, J.S., Haines, M., Doecke, J.D., … Gibson, P.R. (2011). Gluten causes gastrointestinal symptoms in subjects without celiac disease: a double-blind randomized placebo-controlled trial. *Am J Gastroenterol*, 106(3):508-514.

26.   Verdu, E.F., Armstrong, D., & Murray, J.A. (2009). Between celiac disease and irritable bowel syndrome: the "no man's land" of gluten sensitivity. *Am J Gastroenterol*, 104(6):1587-1594.

27.   Carroccio, A., Mansueto, P., Iacono, G., Soresi, M., D'Alcamo, A., Cavataio, F., …Rini, G.B. (2012). Non-celiac wheat sensitivity diagnosed by double-blind placebo-controlled challenge:exploring a new clinical entity. *Am J Gastroenterol*, 107(12):1898-906.

28.   Pietzak, M. (2012). Celiac disease, wheat allergy, and gluten sensitivity: when gluten free is not a fad. *JPEN J Parenter Enteral Nutr*, 36(1 Suppl):68S-75S.

29.   Storrs, C. (2011, Aug 12). Will a gluten-free diet improve your health? CNN.com. Retrieved from *http://www.cnn.com/2011/HEALTH/04/12/gluten.free.diet.improve/index.html*

30.   O'Brien, K. (2011, Nov 25). Should We All Go Gluten-Free? NYTimes.com. Retrieved from *http://www.nytimes.com/2011/11/27/magazine/Should-We-All-Go-Gluten-Free.html?pagewanted=all&r=0*

31.   Hobkirk, K. (2011, Jan 15). How going gluten-free changed my life. Retrieved from *http://kellyhobkirk.com/misc/how-going-gluten-free-changed-my-life/*

32.   Men's Journal. Winning Without Wheat. Retrieved from *http://www.mensjournal.com/health-fitness/nutrition/winning-without-wheat-20120820*

33.   Gluten Free Society. Gluten Free Testimonials. Retrieved from *http://www.glutenfreesociety.org/gluten-free-testimonials/*

34.   annelb (2007, Jun 24). Anne's story. Retrieved from ***http://
www.glutenfreeandbeyond.org/forum/viewtopic.php?t=370***

35.   genieb (2012, May 26). Gluten Free and Loving It!. Retrieved
from ***http://www.glutenfreeandbeyond.org/forum/viewtopic.
php?t=5885***

36.   stegenrae (2010, Dec 15). Finally feeling (almost) "normal".
Retrieved from ***http://www.glutenfreeandbeyond.org/forum/
viewtopic.php?t=5213***

37.   American Academy of Pediatrics (2010). Gastrointestinal
problems common in children with autism. *ScienceDaily*. Retrieved
from ***http://www.sciencedaily.com/releases/2010/05/100502080234.
htm***

38.   Schieve, L.A., Gonzalez, V., Boulet, S.L., Visser, S.N., Rice,
C.E., Braun, K.V., Boyle, C.A. (2012). Concurrent medical conditions
and health care use and needs among children with learning and
behavioral developmental disabilities, National Health Interview
Survey, 2006-2010. *Res Dev Disabil*, 33(2):467-476.

39.   Schieve, L. (2012, Jan 24). Autism and Associated Medical
Conditions. Retrieved from ***http://blog.autismspeaks.org/tag/diarrhea/***

40.   Medical News Today (2012, Mar 1). Some Children With
Autism May Benefit From a Gluten-Free, Casein-Free Diet. *Medical
News Today*. Retrieved from ***http://www.medicalnewstoday.com/
releases/242339.php***

41.   Gorrindo, P., Williams, K.C., Lee, E.B., Walker, L.S.,
McGrew, S.G., & Levitt, P. (2012). Gastrointestinal Dysfunction in
Autism: Parental Report, Clinical Evaluation, and Associated Factors.
Autism Research, 5(2), 101-108.

42.   GFCFDiet.com. Success Stories. Retrieved from ***http://
gfcfdiet.com/successstories.htm***

43.   Elkan, A.C., Sjöberg, B., Kolsrud, B., Ringertz, B., Hafström,

I., & Frosteg⬚rd, J. (2008). Gluten-free vegan diet induces decreased LDL and oxidized LDL levels and raised atheroprotective natural antibodies against phosphorylcholine in patients with rheumatoid arthritis: a randomized study. *Arthritis Res Ther*, 10(2):R34.

44.   Castillo-Ortiz, J.D., Durán-Barragán, S., Sáanchez-Ortiz, A., & Ramos-Remus, C. (2011). [Anti-transglutaminase, antigladin and ultra purified anti-gladin antibodies in patients with a diagnosis of rheumatoid arthritis]. *Reumatol Clin*, 7(1):27-29.

45.   Valentino, R., Savastano, S., Maglio, M., Paparo, F., Ferrar, F., Dorato, M., ... Troncone, R. (2002). Markers of potential coeliac disease in patients with Hashimoto's thyroiditis. *Eur J Endocrinol*, 146(4):479-483.

46.   Füchtenbusch, M., Ziegler, A.G., & Hummel, M. (2004). Elimination of Dietary Gluten and Development of Type 1 Diabetes in High Risk Subjects. *Rev Diabet Stud*, 1(1):39-41.

47.   Ziegler, A.G., Schmid, S., Huber, D., Hummel, M., & Bonifacio, E. (2003). Early infant feeding and risk of developing type 1 diabetes-associated autoantibodies. *JAMA*, 290(13):1721-1728.

48.   Freeman, H.J. (2008). Adult celiac disease followed by onset of systemic lupus erythematosus. *J Clin Gastroenterol*, 42(3):252-255.

49.   Greenblatt, J.M. (2011, May 24). Is Gluten Making You Depressed? *Psychology Today*. Retrieved from ***http://www.psychologytoday.com/blog/the-breakthrough-depression-solution/201105/is-gluten-making-you-depressed***

50.   Ciacci, C., Iavarone, A., Mazzacca, G., & De Rosa, A. (1998). Depressive symptoms in adult coeliac disease. *Scand J Gastroenteol*, 33(3): 247-250.

51.   Medical College of Georgia (2006). Scientists Learn More About How Roughage Keeps You 'Regular'. *ScienceDaily*. Retrieved from ***http://www.sciencedaily.com/releases/2006/08/060823093156.htm***

52.   Sisson, M. (2008, Nov 19). Grain Pain. Retrieved from *http://www.marksdailyapple.com/grain-pain/#axzz21TUVxmGR*

53.   Negri, E., Franceschi, S., Parpinel, M., & La Vecchia, C. (1998). Fiber intake and risk of colorectal cancer. *Cancer Epidemiol Biomarkers Prev*, 7(8):667-671.

54.   Tantamango, Y.M., Knutsen, S.F., Beeson, L., Fraser, G., & Sabate, J. (2011). Association between dietary fiber and incident cases of colon polyps: the adventist health study. *Gastrointest Cancer Res*, 4(5-6):161-167.

55.   Terry, P., Giovannucci, E., Michels, K.B., Bergkvist, L., Hansen, H., Holmberg, L., & Wolk, A. (2001). Fruit, vegetables, dietary fiber, and risk of colorectal cancer. *J Natl Cancer Inst*, 93(7):525-533.

56.   Flood, A., Rastogi, T., Wirfält, E., Mitrou, P.N., Reedy, J., Subar, A.F., … Schatzkin, A. (2008). Dietary patterns as identified by factor analysis and colorectal cancer among middle-aged Americans. *Am J Clin Nutr*, **88(1):176-184.**

57.   Zelman, K.M. (2010, Nov 20). Can Fiber Help Protect Against Cancer? WebMD. Retrieved from *http://www.webmd.com/diet/fiber-health-benefits-11/fiber-cancer?page=1*

58.   Potter, J.D. (1988). Dietary Fiber, Vegetables and Cancer. J Nutr, 118: 1591-1592.

59.   Fukudome, S., & Yoshikawa, M. (1992). Opioid peptides derived from wheat gluten: their isolation and characterization. *FEBS Lett*, 296(1):107-111.

60.   Fukudome, S., & Yoshikawa, M. (1993). Gluten exorphin C. A novel opioid peptide derived from wheat gluten. *FEBS Lett*, 316(1):17-19.

61.   Fukudome, S., & Yoshikawa, M. (1997). Release of opioid peptides, gluten exorphins by the action of pancreatic elastase. *FEBS Lett*, 412(3):475-479.

62.   Smith, M.D. (2002). *Going Against the Grain: How Reducing and Avoiding Grains Can Revitalize Your Health*. New York, NY: McGraw-Hill.

63.   Minich, D.M., & Bland, J.S. (2007). Acid-alkaline balance: role in chronic disease and detoxification. *Altern Ter Health Med*, 13(4):62-65.

64.   Dawson-Hughes, B., Harris, S.S., & Ceglia, L. (2008). Alkaline diets favor lean tissue mass in older adults. *Am J Clin Nutr*, 87(3):662-665.

65.   Khetarpaul, N., & Chauhan, B.M. (2006). Effect of Germination and Fermentation on in vitro Starch and Protein Digestibility of Pearl Millet. *Journal of Food Science*, 55(3):883-884.

66.   Whole Grains Council. Sprouted Whole Grains. Retrieved from ***http://www.wholegrainscouncil.org/whole-grains-101/sprouted-whole-grains***

67.   Abdelrahaman, S.M., Elmaki, H.B., Idris, W.H., Hassan, A.B., Babiker, E.E., & El Tinay, A.H. (2007). Antinutritional factor content and hydrochloric acid extractability of minerals in pearl millet cultivars as affected by germination. *Int J Food Sci Nutr*, 58(1):6-17.

68.   Centeno, C., Viveros, A., Brenes, A., Canales, R., Lozano, A., & dela Cuadra C. (2001). Effect of several germination conditions on total P, phytate P, phytase, and acid phosphatase activities and inositol phosphate esters in rye and barley. *J Agri Food Chem*, 49(7):3208-3215.

69.   Chitra, U., Vimala, V., Singh, U., & Geervani, P. (1995). Variability in phytic acid content and protein digestibility of grain legumes. *Plant Foods Hum Nutr*, 47(2):163-172.

70.   Lajolo, F.M., & Genovese, M.I. (2002). Nutritional significance of lectins and enzyme inhibitors from legumes. *J Agri, Food Chem*, 50(22):6592-6598.

71.   Weder, J.K., & Kahleyss, R. (2003). Reaction of lentil trypsin-

chymotrypsin inhibitors with human and bovine proteinases. *J Agri Food Chem*, 51(27):8045-8050.

72.   Sotelo-López, A., Hernández-Infante, M., Artegaga-Cruz, M.E. (1978). Trypsin inhibitors and hemagglutinins in certain edible leguminosae. *Arch Invest Med (Mex)*, 9(1):1-14.

73.   United States Food and Drug Administration (2012). Bad Bug Book: Foodborne Pathogenic Microorganisms and Natural Toxins Handbook. Retrieved from **http://www. fda.gov/downloads/Food/FoodSafety/FoodborneIllness/ FoodborneIllnessFoodbornePathogensNaturalToxins/BadBugBook/ UCM297627.pdf**

74.   Suarez, F.L., Springfield, J., Furne, J.K., Lohrmann, T.T., Kerr, P.S., & Levitt, M.D. (1999). Gas production in human ingesting a soybean flour derived from beans naturally low in oligosaccharides. *Am J Clin Nutr*, 69(1):135-139.

75.   Carlsson, N.G., Karlsson, H., & Sandberg, A.S. (1992). Determination of oligosaccharides in foods, diets, and intestinal contents by high-temperature gas chromatography and gas chromatography/mass spectrometry. *J Agri Food Chem*, 40(12):2404-2412.

76.   Oboh, H.A., Muzquiz, M., Burbano, C., Cuadrado, C., Pedrosa, M.M., Ayet, G., & Osagie, A.U. (2000). Effect of soaking, cooking and germination on the oligosaccharide content of selected Nigerian legume seeds. *Plant Foods Hum Nutr*, 55(2):97-110.

77.   Food and Agriculture Organization of the United Nations (1990). *Roots, Tubers, Plantains and Bananas.* Retrieved from **http:// www.fao.org/docrep/t0562e/T0562E00.htm#Contents**

78.   Nema, P.K., Ramayya, N., Duncan, E., & Niranjan, K. (2008). Potato glycoalkaloids: formation and strategies for mitigation. *Journal of the Science of Food and Agriculture.* 88(11):1869-1881.

79.   North Carolina Department of Health and Human

Services (2012, Oct 11). N.C. DHHS Confirms First Death from E. coli Infection: State Health Director Urges Precautions to Prevent Infection. Retrieved from *http://www.ncdhhs.gov/pressrel/2012/2012-10-13_first_ecoli_death.htm*

80.   Huffington Post (2012, Dec 3). Salmonella Poisoning From peanuts Killed Jeff Almer's Mother After She Beat Cancer. Retrieved from *http://www.huffingtonpost.com/2012/12/03/salmonella-poisoning-jeff-almer-cancer_n_2235097.html*

81.   Mills, M.R. (2009, Nov 21). The Comparative Anatomy of Eating. Retrieved from *http://www.vegsource.com/news/2009/11/the-comparative-anatomy-of-eating.html*

82.   Greger, Michael (2012, Oct 10). Modern Meat Not Ahead of the Game. Retrieved from *http://nutritionfacts.org/video/modern-meat-not-ahead-of-the-game/*

83.   Dunn, R. (2012, July 23). Human Ancestors Were Nearly All Vegetarians. Retrieved from *http://blogs.scientificamerican.com/guest-blog/2012/07/23/human-ancestors-were-nearly-all-vegetarians/*

84.   Ungar, P.S. & Teaford, M.F. (Eds.) (2002). *Human Diet: It's origin and Evolution*. Westport, CT: Bergin and Garvey.

85.   Understanding Evolution (2007). Got Lactase? Retrieved from *http://evolution.berkeley.edu/evolibrary/news/070401_lactose*

86.   University College London (2009). Milk Drinking Started Around 7,500 Years Ago In Central Europe. *ScienceDaily*. Retrieved from *http://www.sciencedaily.com/releases/2009/08/090827202513.htm*

87.   Ohio State Wexner Medical Center. Lactose Intolerance. Retrieved from *http://medicalcenter.osu.edu/patientcare/healthcare_services/digestive_disorders/lactose_intolerance/Pages/index.aspx*

Chapter 5: The Best Raw Food Diet for Health and Vitality

1.   Foster-Powell, K., Holt, S.H., & Brand-Miller, J.C. (2002).

International table of glycemic index and glycemic load values: 2002. *Am J Clin Nutr*, 76(1):5-56.

2.   American Diabetes Association. Checking Your Blood Glucose. Retrieved from *http://www.diabetes.org/living-with-diabetes/treatment-and-care/blood-glucose-control/checking-your-blood-glucose.html*

3.   Bennett, Don. Q: What causes pain/discomfort when eating sweet fruit like watermelon on an empty stomach? Retrieved from *http://health101.org/art_melon-belly*

4.   University of Georgia (2012). Low oxygen levels could drive cancer growth, research suggest. *ScienceDaily*. Retrieved from *http://www.sciencedaily.com/releases/2012/05/120503194219.htm*

5.   Vaupel, P., & Mayer, A. (2007). Hypoxia in cancer: significance and impact on clinical outcome. *Cancer Matastasis Rev*, 26(2):225-239.

6.   University of California - Riverside (2008). Cancer Treatment: How Eating Fruit And Vegetables Can Improve Cancer Patients' Response To Chemotherapy. *ScienceDaily*. Retrieved from *http://www.sciencedaily.com/releases/2008/10/081022164724.htm*

7.   Lee, C., Raffaghello, L., Brandhorst, S., Safdie, F.M., Bianchi, G., Marth-Montalvo, A., ... Longo, V.D. (2012). Fasting cycles retard growth of tumors and sensitize a range of cancer cell types to chemotherapy. *Sci Transl Med*, 4(124):124ra27.

8.   Safdie, F.M., Dorff, T., Quinn, D., Fontana, L., Wei, M., Lee, C., ... Long, V.D. (2009). Fasting and cancer treatment in humans: A case series report. *Aging (Albany, NY)*, 1(12):988-1007.

9.   Varady, K.A., Roohk, D.J., McEvoy-Hein, B.K., Gaylinn, B.D., Thorner, M.O. & Hellerstein, M.K. (2008). Modified alternate-day fasting regimens reduce cell proliferation rates to a similar extent as daily calorie restriction in mice. *FASEB J*, 22(6):2090-2096.

10.   American Cancer Society (2012). American Cancer Society

Guidelines on Nutrition and Physical Activity for Cancer Prevention. CA: A Cancer Journal for Clinicians. Retrieved from *http://www. cancer.org/acs/groups/cid/documents/webcontent/002577-pdf.pdf*

11.   Huang, D., Dhawan, T., Young, S., Yong, W.H., Boros, L.G., & Heaney, A.P. (2011). Fructose impairs glucose-induced hepatic triglyceride synthesis. *Lipids Health Dis*, 10:20.

12.   Mayo Clinic staff. (2011, Feb 11). Nonalcoholic fatty liver disease: Risk factors. Mayo Clinic. Retrieved from *http://www. mayoclinic.com/health/nonalcoholic-fatty-liver-disease/DS00577/ DSECTION=risk-factors*

13.   Wedro, B. Fatty Liver Disease (NAFLD, NASH). emedicinehealth.com. Retrieved from *http://www.emedicinehealth. com/fatty_liver_disease/article_em.htm*

14.   Arsenault, B.J., Rana, J.S., Stroes, E.S., Després, J.P., Shah, P.K., Kastelein, J.J., … Khaw, K.T. (2009). Beyond low-density lipoprotein cholesterol: respective contributions of non-high-density lipoprotein cholesterol levels, triglycerides, and the total cholesterol/ high-density lipoprotein cholesterol ratio to coronary heart disease risk in apparently healthy men and women. J Am Coll Cardiol, 55(1):35-41.

15.   Wiley-Blackwell (2011). Increasing triglyceride levels linked to greater stroke risk; Study finds higher cholesterol levels only increase risk of stroke in men. *ScienceDaily*. Retrieved from *http:// www.sciencedaily.com/releases/2011/02/110221071523.htm*

16.   New York University Langone Medical Center (2012). Triglyceride levels predict stroke risk in postmenopausal women. *ScienceDaily*. Retrieved from *http://www.sciencedaily.com/ releases/2012/02/120202164536.htm*

17.   Cincinnati Children's Hospital Medical Center (2010). High levels of fructose, trans fats lead to significant liver disease, says study. *ScienceDaily*. Retrieved from *http://www.sciencedaily.com/ releases/2010/06/100622112548.htm*

18.   Ouyang, X., Cirillo, P., Sautin, Y., McCall, S., Bruchette, J.L., Diehl, A.M., ... Abdelmalek, M.F. (2008). Fructose Consumption as a Risk Factor for Non-alcoholic Fatty Liver Disease. J Hepatol, 48(6):993-999.

19.   Teff, K.L., Elliott, S.S., Tschöp, M., Kieffer, T.J., Rader, D., Heiman, M., ... Havel, P.J. (2004). Dietary fructose reduces circulating insulin and leptin, attenuates postprandial suppression of ghrelin, and increases triglycerides in women. *J Clin Endocrinol Metab*, 89(6):2963-2972.

20.   University of Southern California - Health Sciences (2012). Diabetes prevalence 20 percent higher in countries with higher availability of high fructose corn syrup, analysis finds. *ScienceDaily*. Retrieved from *http://www.sciencedaily.com/releases/2012/11/121127111337.htm*

21.   Abdelmalek, M.F., Lazo, M., Horska, A., Bonekamp, S., Lipkin, E.W., Balasubramanyam, A., ... Fatty Liver Subgroup of Look AHEAD Research Group. *Hepatology*, 56(3):952-960.

22.   University of Colorado Denver (2012). Research offers insight to how fructose causes obesity and other illness. *ScienceDaily*. Retrieved from *http://www.sciencedaily.com/releases/2012/02/120227152723.htm*

23.   Wiley (2012). Increased dietary fructose linked to elevated uric acid levels and lower liver energy stores. *ScienceDaily*. Retrieved from *http://www.sciencedaily.com/releases/2012/09/120913104121.htm*

24.   Reuters. (2007, Jan 3). Diet seen to affect liver cancer risk. Retrieved from *http://www.reuters.com/article/2007/01/03/us-liver-cancer-idUSSP14795920070103*

25.   BBC News (2006, Sep 11). Mandarins 'cut liver cancer risk'. Retrieved from *http://news.bbc.co.uk/2/hi/health/5333898.stm*

26.   UC Television (2009, Jul 30). Sugar: The Bitter Truth.

Retrieved from *http://www.youtube.com/watch?v=dBnniua6-oM*

27. WebMD. Candidiasis (Yeast Infection). Retrieved from *http://www.webmd.com/skin-problems-and-treatments/guide/candidiasis-yeast-infection*

28. The Office on Women's Health (2010, May 18). Douching fact sheet. Retrieved from *http://womenshealth.gov/publications/our-publications/fact-sheet/douching.cfm*

29. MedlinePlus (2010, Sep 15). Candida infection of the skin. Retrieved from *http://www.nlm.nih.gov/medlineplus/ency/article/000880.htm*

30. CandidaMD (2011, Jan 12). Candida symptoms. Retrieved from *http://www.candidamd.com/candida/symptoms.html*

31. TheCandidaDiet. Candida Symptoms. Retrieved from *http://www.thecandidadiet.com/candidasymptoms.htm*

32. Perkins, C. Identifying Candida Symptoms. Retrieved from *http://www.holistichelp.net/candida.html*

33. PubMed Health. (2012, Oct 6). Thrush. Retrieved from *http://www.ncbi.nlm.nih.gov/pubmedhealth/PMH0001650/*

34. PubMed Health. (2011, Nov 7). Vaginal yeast infection. Retrieved from *http://www.ncbi.nlm.nih.gov/pubmedhealth/PMH0002480/*

35. Nara, R.O., & Mariner, S.A. (1979). Money By The Mouthful.

36. Appalachian State University (2012). Bananas are as beneficial as sports drinks, study suggests. *ScienceDaily*. Retrieved from *http://www.ncbi.nlm.nih.gov/pmc/articles/PMC1810582/*

37. Young, S.N. (2007). Folate and depression—a neglected problem. *J Psychiatry Neuroschi*, 32(2):80-82.

38. Block, G., Patterson, B., & Subar A. (1992). Fruit, vegetables, and cancer prevention: a review of the epidemiological evidence. Nutr

Cancer, 18(1):1-29.

39.   Cormio, L., De Siati, M., Lorusso, F., Selvaggio, O., Mirabella, L., Sanguedolce, F., & Carrieri, G. (2011). Oral L-citrulline supplementation improves erection hardness in men with mild erectile dysfunction. *Urology*, 77(1):119-122.

40.   Garmyn, M., Ribaya-Mercado, J.D., Russel, R.M., Bhawan, J., & Gilchrest, B.A. (1995). Effect of beta-carotene supplementation on the human sunburn reaction. *Exp Dermatol*, 4(2):104-111.

41.   Köpcke, W., & Krutmann, J. (2008). Protection from sunburn with beta-Carotene—a meta-analysis. *Phtochem Photobiol*, 84(2):284-288.

42.   la Ruche, G., & Césarini, J.P. (1991). Protective effect of oral selenium plus copper associated with vitamin complex on sunburn cell formation in human skin. *Photodermatol Phtoimmunol Photomed*, 8(6):232-235.

43.   Walker, A.F., Bundy, R., Hicks, S.M., & Middleton, R.W. (2002). Bromelain reduces mild acute knee pain and improves well-being in a dose-dependent fashion in an open study of otherwise healthy adults. *Phytomedicine*, 9(8):681-686.

44.   Maurer, H.R. (2001). Bromelain: biochemistry, pharmacology and medical use. *Cell Mol Life Sci*, 58(9):1234-1245.

45.   Graham, D. (2012, Oct 1). Re: Craving greens/salt more than fruits. Retrieved from ***http://www.vegsource.com/talk/raw/messages/100039670.html***

Chapter 6: How to Avoid Nutritional Deficiencies With Raw Foods

1.   Panel on Micronutrients, Subcommittees on Upper Reference Levels of Nutrients and of Interpretation and Use of Dietary Reference Intakes, Standing Committee on the Scientific Evaluation of Dietary Reference Intakes. (2001) *Dietary Reference Intakes for Vitamin A, Vitamin K, Arsenic, Boron, Chromium, Copper, Iodine, Iron, Manganese, Molybdenum, Nickel, Silicon, Vanadium, and Zinc.*

Washington, DC: The National Academies Press.

2.   World Health Organization and Food and Agriculture Organization of the United States. (2004). Vitamin and mineral requirements in human nutrition, 2nd ed. Retrieved from ***http:// whqlibdoc.who.int/publications/2004/9241546123.pdf***

3.   Higdon, J. (2003, Dec). Vitamin A. Linus Pauling Institute. Retrieved from ***http://lpi.oregonstate.edu/infocenter/vitamins/ vitaminA/***

4.   Panel on Dietary Antioxidants and Related Compounds, Subcommittee on Upper Reference Levels of Nutrients, Subcommittee on Interpretation and Uses of DRIs, Standing Committee on the Scientific Evaluation of Dietary Reference Intakes, Food and Nutrition Board, Institute of Medicine. (2000). *Dietary Reference Intakes for Vitamin C, Vitamin E, Selenium, and Carotenoids.* Washington, DC: The National Academies Press.

5.   Jenkinson, A.M., Collins, A.R., Duthie, S.J., Wahle, K.W., & Duthie, G.G. (1999). The effect of increased intakes of polyunsaturated fatty acids and vitamin E on DNA damage in human lymphocytes. *FASEB J*, 13(15):138-142.

6.   Dhanwal, D.K., Dennison, E.M., Harvey, N.C., & Cooper, C. (2011). Epidemiology of hip fracture: Worldwide geographic variation. Indian J Orthop, 45(1):15-22.

7.   Dhanwal, D.K., Cooper, C., & Dennison, E.M. (2010). Geographic Variation in Osteoporotic Hip Fracture Incidence: The Growing Importance of Asian Influences in Coming Decades. *J Osteoporos*, 2010:757102.

8.   Itoh, R., Nishiyama, N., & Suyama. (1998). Dietary protein intake and urinary excretion of calcium: a cross-sectional study in a healthy Japanese population. *Am J Clin Nutr*, 67(3):438-444.

9.   Kerstetter, J.E., & Allen, L.H. (1990). Dietary Protein Increases Urinary Calcium. *J Nutr*, 120:134-136.

10.   Matkovic, V., Ilich, J.Z., Andon, M.B., Hsieh, L.C., Tzagournis, M.A., Lagger, B.J., & Goel, P.K. (1995). Urinary calcium, sodium, and bone mass of young females. *Am J Clin Nutr*, 62(2):417-425.

11.   Ho, S.C., Chen, Y.M., Woo, J.L., Leung, S.S., Lam, T.H., & Janus, E.D. (2001). Sodium is the leading dietary factor associated with urinary calcium excretion in Hong Kong Chinese adults. *Osteoporos Int*, 12(9):723-731.

12.   Dawson-Hughes, B., Harris, S.S., Palermo, N.J., Castaneda-Sceppa, C., Rasmussen, H.M., & Dallal, G.E. (2009). Treatment with Potassium Bicarbonate Lowers Calcium Excretion and Bone Resorption in Older Men and Women. *J Clin Endocrinol Metab*, 94(1):96-102.

13.   Sellmeyer, D.E., Schloetter, M., & Sebastian, A. (2002). Potassium citrate prevents increased urine calcium excretion and bone resorption induced by a high sodium chloride diet. *J Clin Endocrinol Metab*, 87(5):2008-2012.

14.   Criqui, M.H., Langer, R.D., & Reed, D.M. (1989). Dietary alcohol, calcium, and potassium. Independent and combined effects on blood pressure. *Circulation*, 80(3):609-614.

15.   Davis, J.L. (2010, Jun 21). Drink Less for Strong Bones: Tips to avoid getting tipsy. WebMD. Retrieved from ***http://www.webmd. com/osteoporosis/features/alcohol***

16.   Krall, E.A., Dawson-Hughes, B. (1999). Smoking increases bone loss and decreases intestinal calcium absorption. *J Bone Miner Res*, 14(2):215-220.

17.   Need, A.G., Kemp, A., Giles, N., Morris, H.A., Horowitz, M., & Nordin, B.E. (2002). Relationships between intestinal calcium absorption, serum vitamin D metabolites and smoking in postmenopausal women. *Osteoporos Int*, 13(1):83-88.

18.   Klein, R.G., Arnaud, S.B., Gallagher, J.C., Deluca, H.F., &

Riggs, B.L. (1977). Intestinal Calcium Absorption in Exogenous Hypercortisonism: Role of 25-Hydroxyvitamin D and Corticosteroid Dose. *J Clin Invest*, 60(1):253-259.

19.   Massey, L.K., & Whiting, S.J. (1993). Caffeine, urinary calcium, calcium metabolism and bone. *J Nutr*, 123(9):1611-1614.

20.   Massey, L.K., & Berg, T.A. (1985). The effect of dietary caffeine on urinary excretion of calcium, magnesium, phosphorus, sodium, potassium, chloride and zinc in healthy males. *Nutrition Research*, 5(11):1281-1284.

21.   Massey, L.K., & Hollingbery, P.W. (1988). Acute effects of dietary caffeine and aspirin on urinary mineral excretion in pre- and postmenopausal women. *Nutrition Research*, 8(8):845-851.

22.   Macdonald, H.M., & Hardcastle, A.C. (2009). Meta-analysis of the quantity of calcium excretion associated with net acid excretion: caution advised. *Am J Clin Nutr*, 89(3):926-927.

23.   World Health Organization (1996). Trace elements in human nutrition and health. Retrieved from ***http://whqlibdoc.who.int/ publications/1996/9241561734_eng.pdf***

24.   Morck, T.A., Lynch, S.R., & Cook, J.D. (1983). Inhibition of food iron absorption by coffee. *Am J Clin Nutr*, 37(3):416-420.

25.   Hurrell, R.F., Reddy, M., & Cook, J.D. (1999). Inhibition of non-haem iron absorption in man by polyphenolic-containing beverages. *Br J Nutr*, 81(4):289-295.

26.   Zijp, I.M., Korver, O., & Tijburg, L.B., (2000). Effect of tea and other dietary factors on iron absorption. *Crit Rev Food Sci Nutr*, 40(5):371-398.

27.   Penn State (2010). Polyphenol antioxidants inhibit iron absorption. *ScienceDaily*. Retrieved from ***http://www.sciencedaily.com/ releases/2010/08/100823152309.htm***

28.   Cook, J.D., Morck, T.A., Lynch, S.R. (1981). The inhibitory

effect of soy products on nonheme iron absorption in man. *Am J Clin Nutr*, 34(12):2622-2629.

29.   Hallberg, L., Brune, M., & Rossander, L. (1989). Iron absorption in man: ascorbic acid and dose-dependent inhibition by phytate. *Am J Clin Nutr*, 49(1):140-144.

30.   Monsen, E.R. (1988). Iron nutrition and absorption: dietary factors which impact iron bioavailability. *J Am Diet Assoc*, 88(7):786-790.

31.   Hallberg, L., Brune, M., & Rossander-Huthén, L. (1987). Is there a physiological role of vitamin C in iron absorption? *Ann N Y Acad Sci*, 498:324-332.

32.   Sharma, D.C., & Mathur, R. (1995). Correction of anemia and iron deficiency in vegetarians by administration of ascorbic acid. *Indian J Physiol Pharmacol*, 39(4):403-406.

33.   Seshadri, S., Shah, A., & Bhade, S. (1985). Haematologic response of anaemic preschool children to ascorbic acid supplementation. *Hum Nutr Appl Nutr*, 39(2):151-154.

34.   jeramy. (2010, Feb 12). ATTN: Calling all [FEMALE] vegans, raw foodist, and other none meat-eaters.? Retrieved from ***http:// forumhealthcare.org/attn-calling-all-vegans-raw-foodist-and-other-none-meat-eaters-t2137.html***

35.   rootzdawta. (2007, Nov 1). Strict Vegetarians: How long is your period, how heavy, how painful? Retrieved from ***http://www. mothering.com/community/t/782124/strict-vegetarians-how-long-is-your-period-how-heavy-how-painful***

36.   Meneghini, R. (1997). Iron homeostasis, oxidative stress, and DNA damage. *Free Radic Biol Med*, 23(5):783-792.

37.   Kabat, G.C., & Rohan, T.E. (2007). Does excess iron play a role in breast carcinogenesis? An unresolved hypothesis. *Cancer Causes Control*, 18(10):1047-1053.

38.   Qi, L., van Dam, R.M., Rexrode, K., & Hu, F.B. (2007). Heme iron from diet as a risk factor for coronary heart disease in women with type 2 diabetes. *Diabetes Care*, 30(1):101-106.

39.   Ascherio, A., Willet, W.C., Rimm, E.B., Giovannucci, E.L., & Stampfer, M.J. (1994). Dietary iron intake and risk of coronary disease among men. *Circulation*, 89(3):969-974.

40.   Lee, D.H., Anderson, K.E., Harnack, L.J., Folsom, A.R., & Jacobs, D.R. Jr. (2004). Heme Iron, Zinc, Alcohol Consumption, and Colon Cancer: Iowa Women's Health Study. *JNCI J Natl Cancer Inst*, 96(5):403-407.

41.   Standing Committee on the Scientific Evaluation of Dietary Reference Intakes, Food and Nutrition Board, Institute of Medicine. (1997). *Dietary Reference Intakes for Calcium, Phosphorus, Magnesium, Vitamin D, and Fluoride*. Washington, DC: The National Academies Press.

42.   Kemi, V.E., Kärkkäinen, M.U., Rita, H.J., Laaksonen, M.M., Outila, T.A., & Lanberg-Allardt, C.J. (2010). Low calcium:phosphorus ratio in habitual diets affects serum parathyroid hormone concentration and calcium metabolism in healthy women with adequate calcium intake. Br J Nutr, 103(4):561-568.

43.   Panel on Dietary Reference Intakes for Electrolytes and Water, Standing Committee on the Scientific Evaluation of Dietary Reference Intakes. (2005). *Dietary Reference Intakes for Water, Potassium, Sodium, Chloride, and Sulfate*. Washington, DC: The National Academies Press.

44.   Elliott, P., & Brown, I. (2007). Sodium Intakes Around The World. World Health Organization. Retrieved from ***http://www.who. int/dietphysicalactivity/Elliot-brown-2007.pdf***

45.   Almond, C.S., Shin, A.Y., Fortescue, E.B., Mannix, R.C., Wypij, D., Binstadt, B.A., ... Greenes, D.S. (2005). Hyponatremia among runners in the Boston Marathon. *N Engl J Med*, 352(15):1550-1556.

46.   Takahashi, P.Y. (2011, Aug 19). Low blood sodium in older adults: A concern? Mayo Clinic. Retrieved from ***http://www. mayoclinic.com/health/low-blood-sodium/AN00621***

47.   Tobian, L. (1979). Dietary salt (sodium) and hypertension. *The American Journal of Clinical Nutrition*, 32:2659-2662.

48.   World Health Organization (2007). Protein and Amino Acid Requirements in Human Nutrition. Retrieved from ***http://whqlibdoc. who.int/trs/WHO_TRS_935_eng.pdf***

49.   Melhus, H., Michaëlsson, K., Kindmark, A., Bergström, R., Holmberg, L., Mallmin, H., ... Ljunghall, S. (1998). Excessive dietary intake of vitamin A is associated with reduced bone mineral density and increased risk for hip fracture. *Ann Intern Med*, **129(10):770-778.**

50.   A Report of the Standing Committee on the Scientific Evaluation of Dietary Reference Intakes and its Panel on Folate, Other B Vitamins, and Choline and Subcommittee on Upper Reference Levels of Nutrients, Food and Nutrition Board, Institute of Medicine. (1998). *Dietary Reference Intakes for Thiamin, Riboflavin, Niacin, Vitamin B6, Folate, Vitamin B12, Pantothenic Acid, Biotin, and Choline*. Washington, DC: The National Academies Press.

51.   Committee to Review Dietary Reference Intakes for Vitamin D and Calcium, Institute of Medicine. (2011). *Dietary Reference Intakes for Calcium and Vitamin D*. Washington, DC: The National Academies Press.

52.   Morris, M.S., Selhub, J., & Jacques, P.F. (2012). Vitamin B-12 and folate status in relation to decline in scores on the mini-mental state examination in the framingham heart study. *J Am Geriatr Soc*, 60(8):1457-1464.

53.   Scheuerman, A. (2012, Feb 3). Too Much of a Good Thing? Retrieved from ***http://now.tufts.edu/articles/folic-acid-too-much-good-thing***

54.   Morris, M.S., Jacques, P.F., Rosenberg, I.H., & Selhub,

J. (2007). Folate and vitamin B-12 status in relation to anemia, macrocytosis, and cognitive impairment in older Americans in the age of folic acid fortification. Am J Clin Nutr, 85(1):193-200.

55.   Higdon, J. (2001). Manganese. Linus Pauling Institute. Retrieved from *http://lpi.oregonstate.edu/infocenter/minerals/manganese/index.html*

Chapter 7: What About Supplements?

1.   Bee (2012, April 13). Intense stomach pain! after e.v.e.r.y. fruit meal! Retrieved from *http://www.30bananasaday.com/forum/topics/intense-stomach-pain-after-e-v-e-r-y-fruit-meal?*

2.   Bennett, Don. Q: What causes pain/discomfort when eating sweet fruit like watermelon on an empty stomach? Retrieved from *http://health101.org/art_melon-belly*

3.   Pacholok, S.M., & Stuart, J.R. (2005). Could It Be B12? An Epidemic of Misdiagnoses. Sanger, CA: Quill Driver Books/Word Dancer Press.

4.   Kirchheimer, S. (2003, June 18). Vegetarian Diet and B12 Deficiency: Vitamin B12 Deficiency Seen in All Types of Vegetarians. WebMD. Retrieved from *http://www.webmd.com/food-recipes/news/20030618/vegetarian-diet-b12-deficiency*

5.   McBride, J. (2000, Aug 2). B12 Deficiency May Be More Widespread Than Thought. USDA. Retrieved from *http://www.ars.usda.gov/is/pr/2000/000802.htm*

6.   Hokin, B.D., & Butler, T. (1999). Cyanocobalamin (vitamin B-12) status in Seventh-day Adventist ministers in Australia. *Am J Clin Nutr*. 70(3 Suppl):576S-578S.

7.   World Health Organization and Food and Agriculture Organization of the United States. (2004). Vitamin and mineral requirements in human nutrition, 2nd ed. Retrieved from *http://whqlibdoc.who.int/publications/2004/9241546123.pdf*

8.   Herbert, V. (1988). Vitamin B-12: plant sources, requirements, and assay. *Am J Clin Nutr*, 48(3 Suppl):852-858.

9.   Ihobe, H. (1992). Observations on the meat-eating behavior of wild bonobos (*Pan paniscus*) at Wamba, Republic of Zaire. *Primates*, 33(2):247-250.

10.   Rauma, A.L., Törröonen, R., Hänninen, O., & Mykkänen, H. (1995). Vitamin B-12 status of long-term adherents of a strict uncooked vegan diet ("living food diet") is compromised. *J Nutr*, 125(10):2511-2515.

11.   Campbell, C.T. B12 Breakthrough - Missing Nutrient Found in Plants. Retrieved from ***http://www.tcolincampbell.org/courses-resources/article/b12-breakthrough-missing-nutrient-found-in-plants/***

12.   McDougall, J. (2007, Nov). Vitamin B12 Deficiency—the Meat-eaters' Last Stand. *McDougall Newsletter*, 6(11). Retrieved from ***http://www.drmcdougall.com/misc/2007nl/nov/b12.htm***

13.   Norris, J. (2002). Vitamin B12: Are You Getting It? Retrieved from ***http://www.purachlorella.com.br/doc/B122002.pdf***

14.   Mozafar, A. (1994). Enrichment of some B-vitamins in plants with application of organic fertilizers. *Plant and Soil*, 167(2):305-311.

15.   Frost, Robert. All You Need to Know Regarding Vitamin B-12. Retrieved from ***http://health.groups.yahoo.com/group/notmilk/message/4031***

16.   Carmel, R., & Bernstein, G.S. (1984). Transcobalamin II in human seminal plasma. *J Clin Invest*, 73(3):868-872.

17.   Norman Clinical Laboratory. Serum b12 Assay. Retrieved from ***http://www.b12.com/uMMA.htm***

18.   News-Medical.net (2004, Oct 28). Test used to diagnose B12 deficiency may be inadequate. Retrieved from ***http://www.news-medical.net/news/2004/10/28/5908.aspx***

19.   Oh, R.C., & Brown, D.L. (2003). Vitamin B12 Deficiency. *Am Fam Physician*, 67(5):979-986.

20.   Higdon, J. (2003). Vitamin B12. Linua Pauling Institute. Retrieved from ***http://lpi.oregonstate.edu/infocenter/vitamins/ vitaminB12/index.html***

21.   Braun-Falco, O., & Lincke, H. (1976). [The problem of vitamin B6/B12 acne. A contribution on acne medicamentosa (author's transl)]. *MMW Munch Med Wochenschr*, 118(6):155-160.

22.   Scheretz, E.F. (1991). Acneiform eruption due to "megadose" vitamins B6 and B12. *Cutis*, 48(2):119-120.

23.   Jansen, T., Romiti, R., Kreuter, A., & Altmeyer, P. (2001). Rosacea fulminans triggered by high-dose vitamins B6 and B12. *J Eur Acad Dermatol Venereol*, 15(5):484-485.

24.   Norris, J. Recommendations. Retrieved from ***http:// veganhealth.org/b12/rec***

25.   Norris, J. Alternatives to Cyanocobalamin: Methylcobalamin & Dibencozide. Retrieved from ***http://veganhealth.org/b12/ noncyanob12***

26.   Davis, D.R., Epp, M.D., & Riordan, H.D. (2004). Changes in USDA food composition data for 43 garden crops, 1950 to 1999. *J Am Coll Nutr*, 23(6):669-682.

27.   Mayer, A.M. (1997). Historical changes in the mineral content of fruits and vegetables. *British Food Journal*, 99(6):207-211.

28.   Dangour, A.D., Dodhia, S.K., Hayter, A., Allen, E., Lock, K., & Uauy, R. (2009). Nutritional quality of organic foods: a systemic review. *Am J Clin Nutr*, 90(3):680-685.

29.   Smith-Spangler, C., Brandea, M.L., Hunter, G.E., Bavinger, J.C., Pearson, M., Eschbach, P.J., … Bravata, D.M. (2012). Are organic foods safer or healthier than conventional alternatives?: a systematic review. *Ann Intern Med*, 157(5):348-366.

30.   Electronic Code of Federal Regulations. Title 7: Agriculture - Part 205—National Organic Program. United States Government Printing Office. Retrieved from ***http://www.ecfr.gov/cgi-bin/text-idx?c=ecfr&SID=96903fddb47d9f10a804350e301e369e&rgn=div5&view=text&node=7:3.1.1.9.32&idno=7***

31.   Panel on Micronutrients, Subcommittees on Upper Reference Levels of Nutrients and of Interpretation and Use of Dietary Reference Intakes, Standing Committee on the Scientific Evaluation of Dietary Reference Intakes. (2001) *Dietary Reference Intakes for Vitamin A, Vitamin K, Arsenic, Boron, Chromium, Copper, Iodine, Iron, Manganese, Molybdenum, Nickel, Silicon, Vanadium, and Zinc.* Washington, DC: The National Academies Press.

32.   Panel on Dietary Antioxidants and Related Compounds, Subcommittee on Upper Reference Levels of Nutrients, Subcommittee on Interpretation and Uses of DRIs, Standing Committee on the Scientific Evaluation of Dietary Reference Intakes, Food and Nutrition Board, Institute of Medicine. (2000). *Dietary Reference Intakes for Vitamin C, Vitamin E, Selenium, and Carotenoids.* Washington, DC: The National Academies Press.

33.   A Report of the Standing Committee on the Scientific Evaluation of Dietary Reference Intakes and its Panel on Folate, Other B Vitamins, and Choline and Subcommittee on Upper Reference Levels of Nutrients, Food and Nutrition Board, Institute of Medicine. (1998). *Dietary Reference Intakes for Thiamin, Riboflavin, Niacin, Vitamin B6, Folate, Vitamin B12, Pantothenic Acid, Biotin, and Choline.* Washington, DC: The National Academies Press.

34.   Brøndum,-Jacobsen, P., Been, M., Jensen, G.B., & Nordestgaard, B.G. (2012). 25-hydroxyvitamin d levels and risk of ischemic heart disease, myocardial infarction, and early death: population-based study and meta-analyses of 18 and 17 studies. *Arterioscler Thromb Vasc Biol*, 32(11):2794-2802.

35.   Ullah, M.I., Uwaifo, G.I., Nicholas, W.C., & Koch, C.A. (2010). Does Vitamin D Deficiency Cause Hypertension? Current

Evidence from Clinical Studies and Potential Mechanisms. *International Journal of Endocrinology*, 2010:579640.

36.   Hultin, H., Edfeldt, K. Sundborn, M., & Hellman, P. (2010). Left-shifted relation between calcium and parathyroid hormone in obesity. *J Clin Endocrinol Metb*, 95(8):3973-3981.

37.   Vieira, V.M., Hart, J.E., Webster, T.F., Weinberg, J., Puett, R., Laden, F., ... Karlson, E.W. (2010). Association between Residences in U.S. Northern Latitudes and Rheumatoid Arthritis: A Spatial Analysis of the Nurses' Health Study. *Environ Health Perspect*, 118(7):957-961.

38.   Llewellyn, D.J., Lang, I.E., Langa, K.M., Muniz-Terrera, G., Phillips, C.L., Cherubini, A., ... Melzer, D. (2010). Vitamin D and risk of cognitive decline in elderly persons. *Arch Intern Med*, 170(13):1135-1141.

39.   Grant, W.B. (2002). An estimate of premature cancer mortality in the U.S. due to inadequate doses of solar ultraviolet-B radiation. *Cancer*, 94(6):1867-1875.

40.   Moan, J., Porojnicu, A.C., Dahlback, A., & Setlow, R.B. (2008). Addressing the health benefits and risks, involving vitamin D or skin cancer, of increased sun exposure. *Proc Natl Acad Sci U S A*, 105(2):668-673.

41.   Committee to Review Dietary Reference Intakes for Vitamin D and Calcium, Institute of Medicine. (2011). *Dietary Reference Intakes for Calcium and Vitamin D*. Washington, DC: The National Academies Press.

42.   Bischoff-Ferraro, H.A., Giovannucci, E., Willett, W.C., Dietrich, T., & Dawson-Hughes, B. (2006). Estimation of optimal serum concentrations of 25-hydroxyvitamin D for multiple health outcomes. *Am J Clin Nutr*, 84(1):18-28.

43.   Bischoff-Ferrari, H.A., Shao, A., Dawson-Hughes, B., Hathcock, J., Giovannucci, E., & Willett, W.C. (2010). Benefit-risk

assessment of vitamin D supplementation. *Osteoporos Int*, 21(7):1121-1132.

44.   Bischoff-Ferrari, H.A., Dawson-Hughes, B., Staehelin, H.B., Orav, J.E., Stuck, A.E., Theiler, R. ... Henschkowshi, J. (2009). Fall prevention with supplemental and active forms of vitamin D: a meta-analysis of randomised controlled trials. *BMJ*, 339:b3692.

45.   Bischoff-Ferrari, H.A., Willett, W.C., Wong, J.B., Stuck, A.E., Staehelin, H.B., Orav, E.J., ... Henschkowski, J. (2009). Prevention of nonvertebral fractures with oral vitamin D and dose dependency: a meta-analysis of randomized controlled trials. *Arch Intern Med*, 169(6):551-561.

46.   Holick, M.F. (2010). *The Vitamin D Solution: A 3-Step Strategy to Cure Our Most Common Health Problems*. New York, NY: Penguin Group.

47.   Bischoff-Ferrari, H., & Willett, W. Comment on the IOM Vitamin D and Calcium Recommendations. Harvard School of Public Health. Retrieved from ***https://www.hsph.harvard.edu/nutritionsource/what-should-you-eat/vitamin-d-fracture-prevention/index.html***

48.   Heaney, R.P. (2005). The Vitamin D requirement in health and disease. *J Steroid Biochem Mol Biol*, 97(1-2):13-19.

49.   Garland, C.F., Gorham, E.D., Mohr, S.B., & Garland, F.C. (2009). Vitamin D for cancer prevention: global perspective. *Ann Epidemiol*, 19(7):468-483.

50.   Pittas, A.G., Nelson, J., Mitri, J., Hillmann, W., Garganta, C., Nathan, D., ... Diabetes Prevention Program Research Group. (2011). Vitamin D Status and Progression to Diabetes in Patients at Risk for Diabetes: An Ancillary Analysis in the Diabetes Prevention Program Randomized Controlled Trial. DiabetesPro.

51.   Johns Hopkins Medicine (2012). Low vitamin D levels linked to more severe multiple sclerosis symptoms. *ScienceDaily*. Retrieved

from *http://www.sciencedaily.com/releases/2012/10/121002091755.htm*

52.   Davidson, M.B., Duran, P., Lee, M.L., & Friedman, T.C. (2012). High-Dose Vitamin D Supplementation in People With Prediabetes and Hypovitaminosis D. *Diabetes Care.* [Epub ahead of print]

53.   Jørgensen, D.H.L., Christensen, J., Schwarz, P., Heegaard, A.M., & Lind, B. (2012). A Reverse J-Shaped Association of All-Cause Mortality with Serum 25-Hydroxyvitamin D in General Practice, the CopD Study. *The Journal of Clinical Endocrinology & Metabolism*, 87(8):2644-2652.

54.   Vieth, R., (2011). Why the minimum desirable serum 25-hydroxyvitamin D level should be 75 nmol/L (30 ng/ml). *Best Prac Res Clin Endocrinol Metab*, 25(4):681-691.

55.   Luxwolda, M.F., Kuipers, R.S., Keman, I.P., Janneke Dijck-Brouwer, D.A., & Muskiet, F.A. (2012). Traditionally living populations in East Africa have a mean serum 25-hydroxyvitamin D concentration of 115 nmol/l. *Br J Nutr*, 108(9):1557-1561.

56.   Matsuoka, L.Y., Wortsman, J., Hanifan, N., & Holick, M.F. (1988). Chronic sunscreen use decreases circulating concentrations of 25-hydroxyvitamin D. A preliminary study. *Arch Dermatol*, 124(12):1802-1804.

57.   Matsuoka, L.Y., Ide, L., Wortsman, J., MacLaughlin, J.A., & Holick, M.F. (1987). Sunscreens suppress cutaneous vitamin D3 synthesis. *J Clin Endocrinol Metab*, 64(6):1165-1168.

58.   Holick, M.F. (2012). Evidence-based D-bate on health benefits of vitamin D revisited. *Dermato Endocrinology*, 4(2):183-190.

59.   Fudge, T. (2009, June 3). Cancer Specialist: Sun Exposure Does Not Cause Melanoma. KPBS. Retrieved from *http://www.kpbs.org/news/2009/jun/03/sun-exposure-does-not-cause-melanoma/*

60.	Elwood, J.M., & Jopson, J. (1997). Melanoma and sun exposure: an overview of published studies. *Int J Cancer*, 73(2):198-203.

61.	Kennedy, C., Bajdik, C.D., Willemze, R., De Gruijl, F.R., Bouwes Bavinck, J.N., & Leiden Skin Cancer Study. (2003). The influence of painful sunburns and lifetime sun exposure on the risk of actinic keratoses, seborrheic warts, melanocytic nevi, atypical nevi, and skin cancer. *J Invest Dermatol*, 120(6):1087-1093.

62.	Garland, F.C., White, M.R., Garland, C.F., Shaw, E. & Gorham, E.D. (1990). Occupational sunlight exposure and melanoma in the U.S. Navy. *Arch Environ Health*, 45(5):261-267.

63.	la Ruche, G., & Césarini, J.P. (1991). Protective effect of oral selenium plus copper associated with vitamin complex on sunburn cell formation in human skin. *Photodermatol Phtoimmunol Photomed*, 8(6):232-235.

64.	Köpcke, W., & Krutmann, J. (2008). Protection from sunburn with beta-Carotene—a meta-analysis. *Photochem Photobiol*, 84(2):284-288.

65.	Black, H.S., Herd, J.A., Goldberg, L.H., Wolf, J.E. Jr., Thornby, J.I., Rosen, T., ... et. al. (1994). Effect of a low-fat diet on the incidence of actinic keratosis. *N Engl J Med*, 330(18):1272-1275.

66.	United States Environmental Protection Agency. Monthly Average UV Index. Retrieved from ***http://www.epa.gov/sunwise/uvimonth.html***

67.	Vitamin D Council. (2011, Sep 21). UVB exposure: sunlight and indoor tanning. Retrieved from ***http://www.vitamindcouncil.org/about-vitamin-d/how-to-get-your-vitamin-d/uvb-exposure-sunlight-and-indoor-tanning/***

68.	Lagunova, Z., Porojnicu, A.C., Lindberg, F., Hexeberg, S., & Moan, J. (2009). The Dependency of Vitamin D Status on Body Mass Index, Gender, Age and Season. *Anticancer Research*, 29(9):3713-3720.

69.   Wortsman, J., Matsuoka, L.Y., Chen, T.C., Lu, Z., & Holick, M.F. (2000). Decreased bioavailability of vitamin D in obesity. *Am J Clin Nutr*, 72(3):690-693.

70.   Wasserman, R.H. (2004). Vitamin D and the dual processes of intestinal calcium absorption. *J Nutr*, 134(11)3137-3139.

71.   Heaney, R.P., Dowell, M.S., Hale, C.A., Bendich, A. (2003). Calcium absorption varies within the reference range for serum 25-hydroxyvitamin D. *J Am Coll Nutr*, 22(2):142-146.

72.   Armas, L.A., Hollis, B.W., & Heaney, R.P. (2004). Vitamin D2 is much less effective than vitamin D3 in humans. *J Clin Endocrinol Metab*, 89(11):5387-5391.

73.   Trang, H.M., Cole, D.E., Rubin, L.A., Pierratos, A., Siu, S., & Vieth, R. (1998). Evidence that vitamin D3 increases serum 25-hydroxyvitamin D more efficiently than does vitamin D2. *Am J Clin Nutr*, 68(4):854-858.

74.   Heaney, R.P., Recker, R.R., Grote, J., Horst, R.L., & Armas, L.A. (2011). Vitamin D(3) is more potent than vitamin D(2) in humans. *J Clin Endocrinol Metab*, 96(3):E447-452.

75.   Holick, M.F., Biancuzzo, R.M., Chen, T.C., Klein, E.K., Young, A., Bibuld, D., ... Tannenbaum, A.D. (2008). Vitamin D2 is as effective as vitamin D3 in maintaining circulating concentrations of 25-hydroxyvitamin D. *J Clin Endocrinol Metab*, 93(3):677-681.

76.   Boston University Medical Center (2009). Weekly And Biweekly Vitamin D2 Prevents Vitamin D Deficiency. *ScienceDaily*. Retrieved from ***http://www.sciencedaily.com/releases/2009/10/091026161850.htm***

77.   Norris, J. (2011, Sep). Bones, Vitamin D, and Calcium. Retrieved from ***http://www.veganhealth.org/articles/bones***

78.   Holick, M.F., Binkley, N.C., Bischoff-Ferrari, H.A., Gordon, C.M., Hanley, D.A., Heaney, R.P., ... Endocrine Society (2011).

Evaluation, treatment, and prevention of vitamin D deficiency: an Endocrine Society clinical practice guideline. *J Clin Endocrinol Metab*, 96(7):1911-1930.

79.   UC Television (2009, Mar 5). Vitamin D and Prevention of Chronic Disease. Retrieved from ***http://www.youtube.com/watch?v=Cq1t9WqOD-0***

80.   Mastaglia, S.R., Mautalen, C.A., Parisi, M.S., & Oliveri, B. (2006). Vitamin D2 dose required to rapidly increase 25OHD levels in osteoporotic women. *Eur J Clin Nutr*, 60(5):681-687.

81.   Niramitmahapanya, S., Harris, S.S., & Dawson-Hughes, B. (2011). Type of dietary fat is associated with the 25-hydroxyvitamin D3 increment in response to vitamin D supplementation. J Clin Endocrinol Metab, 96(10):3170-3174.

82.   Mulligan, G.B. (2010). Taking vitamin D with the largest meal improves absorption and results in higher serum levels of 25-hydroxyvitamin D. *J Bone Miner Res*, 25(4):928-930.

83.   Zeratsky, K. (2012, Mar 20). Vitamin D toxicity: What if you get too much? Mayo Clinic. Retrieved from ***http://www.mayoclinic.com/health/vitamin-d-toxicity/AN02008***

84.   Mayo Clinic Staff (2011, May 26). Hypercalcemia: Complications. Mayo Clinic. Retrieved from ***http://www.mayoclinic.com/health/hypercalcemia/DS00976/DSECTION=complications***

Chapter 8: Health Isn't Just About What You Eat

1.   Committee on Sleep Medicine and Research. (2006). *Sleep Disorders and Sleep Deprivation: An Unmet Public Health Problem.* Washington, DC: The National Academies Press.

2.   Shlisky, J.D., Hartman, T.J., Kris-Etherton, P.M., Rogers, C.J., Sharkey, N.A., & Nockols-Richardson, S.M. (2012). Partial sleep deprivation and energy balance in adults: an emerging issue for consideration by dietetics practitioners. J Acad Nutr Diet, 112(11):1785-1797.

3.   Uppsala University (2012). Lack of sleep makes your brain hungry. *ScienceDaily*. Retrieved from *http://www.sciencedaily.com/releases/2012/01/120118111740.htm*

4.   Knutson, K.L. (2012). Does inadequate sleep play a role in vulnerability to obesity? *Am J Hum Biol*, 24(3):361-371.

5.   Matthews, K.A., Dahl, R.E., Owens, J.F., Lee, L., & Hall, M. (2012). Sleep duration and insulin resistance in healthy black and white adolescents. *Sleep*, 35(10):1353-1358.

6.   The Endocrine Society (2010). One sleepless night can induce insulin resistance in healthy people. *ScienceDaily*. Retrieved from *http://www.sciencedaily.com/releases/2010/05/100505091632.htm*

7.   Preidt, R. (2012, Oct 2). Poor Sleep in Teen Years Linked to Heart Risks in Adults. Medline Plus. Retrieved from *http://www.nlm.nih.gov/medlineplus/news/fullstory_129841.html*

8.   Centers for Disease Control and Prevention. (2009, Aug 31). Are You Getting Enough Sleep? Retrieved from *http://www.cdc.gov/partners/Archive/Sleep/index.html*

9.   National Sleep Foundation. How Much Sleep Do We Really Need? Retrieved from *http://www.sleepfoundation.org/article/how-sleep-works/how-much-sleep-do-we-really-need*

10.   Harvard School of Public Health (2012). Weight training linked to reduced risk of type 2 diabetes. *ScienceDaily*. Retrieved from *http://www.sciencedaily.com/releases/2012/08/120806161816.htm*

11.   Pitsavos, C., Panagiotakos, D., Weinem, M., & Stefanadis, C. (2006). Diet, Exercise and the Metabolic Syndrome. *Rev Diabet Stud*, 3(3):118-126.

12.   Washington University School of Medicine (2010). Consistent exercise associated with lower risk of colon cancer death. *ScienceDaily*. Retrieved from *http://www.sciencedaily.com/releases/2010/12/101230172419.htm*

13.   McCullough, L.E., Eng, S.M., Bradshaw, P.T., Cleveland, R.J., Teitelbaum, S.L., Neugut, A.I., & Gammon, M.D. (2012). Fat or fit: the joint effects of physical activity, weight gain, and body size on breast cancer risk. *Cancer*, 118(19):4860-4868.

14.   American Academy of Neurology (2007). Exercise May Lower Risk For Parkinson's Disease. *ScienceDaily*. Retrieved from ***http:// www.sciencedaily.com/releases/2007/04/070423185735.htm***

15.   Weiss, A., Suzuki, T., Bean, J. & Fielding, R.A. (2000). High intensity strength training improves strength and functional performance after stroke. *Am J Phys Med Rehabil*, 79(4):369-376.

16.   Brooks, N., Layne, J.E., Gordon, P.L., Roubenoff, R., Nelson, M.E., & Castaneda-Sceppa, C. (2006). Strength training improves muscle quality and insulin sensitivity in Hispanic older adults with type 2 diabetes. *Int J Med Sci*, 4(1):19-27.

17.   Craft, L.L., & Perna, F.M. (2004). The Benefits of Exercise for the Clinically Depressed. *Prim Care Companion J Clin Psychiatry*, 6(3):104-111.

18.   Krieger, J.W. (2009). Single versus multiple sets of resistance exercise: a meta-regression. *J Strength Cond Res*, 23(6):1890-1901.

19.   Wolfe, B.L., LeMura, L.M., & Cole, P.J. (2004). Quantitative analysis of single- vs. multiple-set programs in resistance training. *J Strength Cond Res*, 18(1):35-47.

20.   Munn, J, Herbert, R.D., Hancock, M.J., Gandevia, S.C. (2005). Resistance training for strength: effect of number of sets and contraction speed. *Med Sci Sports Exerc*, 37(9):1622-1626.

21.   Kerr, D., Morton, A., Dick, I., & Prince, R. (1996). Exercise effects on bone mass in postmenopausal women are site-specific and load-dependent. *J Bone Miner Res*, 11(2):218-225.

22.   Taaffe, D.R., Pruitt, L., Pyka, G., Guido, D., & Marcus, R. (1996). Comparative effects of high- and low-intensity resistance

training on thigh muscle strength, fiber area, and tissue composition in elderly women. *Clin Physiol*, 16(4):381-392.

23.   Guimarães, G.V., Ciolac, E.G., Carvalho, V.O., D'Avila, V.M., Bortolotto, L.A. & Bocchi, E.A. (2010). Effects of continuous vs. interval exercise training on blood pressure and arterial stiffness in treated hypertension. *Hypertens Res*, 33(6):627-632.

24.   Helgerud, J., Høydal, K., Wang, E., Karlsen, T., Berg, P., Bjerkaas, M., ... Hoff, J. (2007). Aerobic high-intensity intervals improve VO2max more than moderate training. *Med Sci Sports Exerc*, 39(4):665-671.

25.   University of Copenhagen (2009). Runners: Train less and be faster. *ScienceDaily*. Retrieved from ***http://www.sciencedaily.com/releases/2009/11/091111122026.htm***

26.   Gibala, M.J., Little, J.P., van Essen, M., Wilkin, G.P., Burgomaster, K.A., Safdar, Adeel, ... Tarnopolsky, M.A. (2006). Short-term sprint interval *versus* traditional endurance training: similar initial adaptations in human skeletal muscle and exercise performance. *J Physiol*, 575(Pt 3):901-911.

27.   Finn, C. (2001, Mar). Effects of High-Intensity Intermittent Training on Endurance Performance. Sportscience, 5(1). Retrieved from ***http://www.sportsci.org/jour/0101/cf.htm***

28.   Tjønna, A.E., Lee, S.J., Rognmo, Ø, Stølen, T.O., Bye, A., Haram, P.M., ... Wisløff, U. (2008). Aerobic interval training versus continuous moderate exercise as a treatment for the metabolic syndrome: a pilot study. *Circulation*, 118(4):346-354.

29.   Burgomaster, K.A., Hughes, S.C., Heigenhauser, G.J., Bradwell, S.N., & Gibala, M.J. (2005). Six sessions of sprint interval training increases muscle oxidative potential and cycle endurance capacity in humans. *J Appl Physiol*, 98(6):1985-1990.

30.   Rakobowchuk, M., Tanguay, S., Burgomaster, K.A., Howarth, K.R., Gibala, M.J., & MacDonald, M.J. (2008). Sprint interval

and traditional endurance training induce similar improvements in peripheral arterial stiffness and flow-mediated dilation in healthy humans. *Am J Physiol Regul Integr Comp Physiol*, 295(1):R236-242.

31.   Hobson, K. (2011, Jun 28). To Heal a Heart, Train Harder: Not Just for Athletes, Intense Exercise Replaces Slow, Steady Regimen. The Wall Street Journal. Retrieved from *http://online.wsj.com/article/SB10001424052702303627104576411633459906142.html*

32.   Boutcher, S.H. (2011). High-intensity intermittent exercise and fat loss. J Obes, 2011:868305.

33.   Hood, M.S., Little, J.P., Tarnopolsky, M.A., Myslik, F., & Gibala, M.J. (2011). Low-volume interval training improves muscle oxidative capacity in sedentary adults. *Med Sci Sports Exerc*, 43(10):1849-1856.

34.   Boudou, P., Sobngwi, E., Mauvais-Jarvis, F., Vexiau, P., & Gautier, J.F. (2003). Absence of exercise-induced variations in adiponectin levels despite decreased abdominal adiposity and improved insulin sensitivity in type 2 diabetic men. *Eur J Endocrinol*, 149(5):421-424.

35.   Babraj, J.A., Vollaard, N.B.J., Keast, C., Guppy, F.M., Cottrell, G., & Timmons, J.A. (2009). Extremely short duration high intensity interval training substantially improves insulin action in young healthy males. *BMC Endocr Disord*, 9:3.

36.   Talanian, J.L., Galloway, S.D., Heigenhauser, G.J., Bonen, A., & Spriet, L.L. (2007). Two weeks of high-intensity aerobic interval training increases the capacity for fat oxidation during exercise in women. *J Appl Physiol*, 102(4):1439-1447.

37.   Perry, C.G., Heigenhauser, G.J., Bonen, A., & Spriet, L.L. (2008). High-intensity aerobic interval training increases fat and carbohydrate metabolic capacities in human skeletal muscle. *Appl Physiol Metab*, 33(6):1112-1123.

38.   Tremblay, A, Simoneau, J.A., & Bouchard, C. (1994). Impact of exercise intensity on body fatness and skeletal muscle metabolism. *Metabolism*, 43(7):814-818.

39.   Heydari, M., Freund, J., & Bouchar, S.H. (2012). The effect of high-intensity intermittent exercise on body composition of overweight young males. *J Obes*, 2012:480467.

40.   Vella, C.A., & Kravitz, L. Exercise After-Burn: Research Update. Retrieved from ***http://www.unm.edu/~lkravitz/Article%20 folder/epocarticle.html***

41.   Schuenke, M.D., Mikat, R.P., & McBride, J.M. (2002). Effect of an acute period of resistance exercise on excess post-exercise oxygen consumption: implications for body mass management. *Eur J Appl, Physiol*, 86(5):411-417.

42.   Elsevier (2012). Excessive endurance training can be too much of a good thing, research suggests. *ScienceDaily*. Retrieved from ***http:// www.sciencedaily.com/releases/2012/06/120604093108.htm***

43.   European Society of Cardiology (2012). Endurance exercise linked to damage in right ventricle of heart. *ScienceDaily*. Retrieved from ***http://www.sciencedaily.com/releases/2011/12/111207000759. htm***

44.   Burrows, M., Nevill, A.M., Bird, S., & Simpson, D. (2003). Physiological factors associated with low bone mineral density in female endurance runners. *Br J Sports Med*, 37(1):67-71.

45.   Hinton, P. (2007, Oct 15). Study Shows Some Athletic Men May Risk Low Bone Density. Retrieved from ***http://munews. missouri.edu/news-releases/2007/1015-hinton-osteopenia.php***

46.   Hetland, M.L., Haarbo, J., Christiansen, C. (1993). Low bone mass and high bone turnover in male long distance runners. *J Clin Endocrinol Metab*, 77(3):770-775.

47.   Warren, M.P. (1999). Health issues for women athletes:

exercise-induced amenorrhea. *J Clin Endocrinol Metab*, 84(6):1892-1896.

48.   Sapolsky, R.M. (2004). *Why Zebras Don't Get Ulcers* (3rd ed.). New York, NY: Henry Holt and Company.

Made in the USA
Lexington, KY
13 March 2014